Coping with Low Vision

Coping with Aging Series

Series Editor
John C. Rosenbek, Ph.D.
Chief, Speech Pathology and Audiology Services
William S. Middleton Memorial Hospital
Madison, Wisconsin

Medical Editor
Molly Carnes, M.D.
Department of Medicine and Institute on Aging
University of Wisconsin
Madison, Wisconsin

Chief, Geriatrics Section
William S. Middleton Memorial Hospital
Madison, Wisconsin

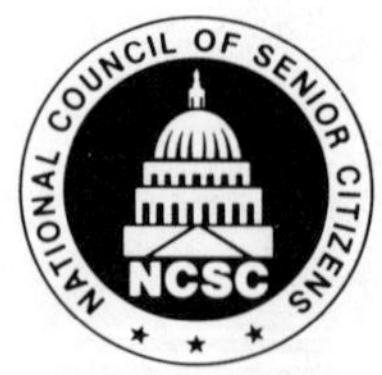

Published in Cooperation with
the National Council of Senior Citizens

Coping with Low Vision

Marshall E. Flax, M.S.
Don J. Golembiewski, M.A.
Bette L. McCaulley, R.N., M.S.

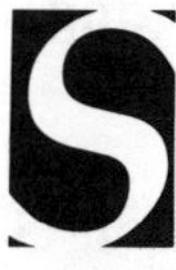

SINGULAR PUBLISHING GROUP, INC.
SAN DIEGO, CALIFORNIA

Illustrations by
Betsy True

Published by Singular Publishing Group, Inc.
4284 41st Street
San Diego, California 92105-1197

Typeset in 14/18 Times by CFW Graphics
Printed in the United States of America by McNaughton & Gunn

Library of Congress Cataloging-in-Publication Data

Flax, Marshall E.
Coping with low vision / Marshall E. Flax, Don J. Golembiewski Bette L. McCaulley.
p. cm. — (Coping with aging series)
Includes index.
ISBN 1-879105-71-3
1. Low vision—Popular works. I. Golembiewski, Don J. II. McCaulley, Bette, L. III. Title. IV. Series.
RE91.F53 1993
362.4′1—dc20 92-31826
CIP

❖ Table of Contents

❖ Foreword

The books in the *Coping with Aging Series* are written for men and women coping with the challenges of aging, and for their families and other caregivers. The authors are all experienced practitioners: doctors, nurses, social workers, psychologists, pharmacists, nutritionists, audiologists, physical and occupational therapists, low vision therapists, rehabilitation teachers, and speech-language pathologists.

The topics of individual volumes are as varied as are the challenges that aging may bring. These include: hearing loss, low vision, depression, sexual dysfunction, immobility, intellectual impairment, language impairment, speech impairment, swallowing impairment, death and dying, bowel and bladder incontinence, stress of caregiving, giving up independence, medications, and stroke. The volumes themselves, however, share common features. Foremost, they are practical, jargon-free, and responsible. Each contains professionally valid information translated into language people who are not health care providers can understand. Each contains useful advice and sections to help readers decide how they are doing and whether they need to do more, do less, or do something different. Each includes lists of services, suppliers, and additional readings. Each provides evidence that no single person need cope alone.

None of the volumes can substitute for appropriate professional health care. However, when combined with the care, instruction, and counseling that health care providers supply, they make coping with aging easier.

America is greying at the same time its treasury is inadequate to meet its population's needs. Thus the *Coping with Aging Series* offers help for people who need and want to help themselves.

This volume, *Coping with Low Vision,* is written to answer the many questions that arise when you or a family member is diagnosed as having low vision. The authors provide useful information on low vision along with many helpful suggestions that will allow you or your family member to cope with this condition. There are many things that can be done to help you continue with your daily activities that may be affected by low vision, and you will find these solutions in this book.

John C. Rosenbek, Ph.D.
Series Editor

Molly Carnes, M.D.
Medical Editor

❖ Preface

Welcome to *Coping with Low Vision,* a self-help guide and resource manual for partially sighted people and their families. This is not a book with lots of charts, graphs, and footnotes to be used primarily for research or academic purposes. Rather, it is a "hands-on" book about how to cope with real problems in a real world. It is our hope that the information you are about to read will help you to live a fuller and more independent life.

How did you first hear about low vision? Most people have never heard of the term until they hear it from an eye doctor. He or she may explain why regular glasses won't help you see any better and use the term "low vision." In fact, the whole concept of having an eye condition that is not totally blinding but cannot be corrected by regular glasses is new to most people. Many people are unaware of the extent of the problem or that there are a number of professional services available to help them cope with their situation. Sadly, people with low vision often spend months or years learning a little here and a little there; following up on stories they have been told by well-meaning friends and relatives about treatments, cures, and special magnifying aids; and slowly restricting their lives because they can't see well and they don't know what to do about it.

Coping With Low Vision is directed to the largest group affected by vision impairment, people in their 60s and older. The main concerns of this group usually are:

1. Will I go completely blind?
2. How will I take care of myself on a daily basis independently and with dignity?
3. How can I see well enough to manage my financial affairs?
4. How will I get around?
5. How can I keep from becoming a burden to my family?

The answers to each of these questions will vary for each individual, but, regardless of the extent of vision loss, there is always something that can be done to help you cope.

Having low vision causes people to have certain difficulties in many common daily living activities. In this book, you will find solutions to some of the most common questions and concerns people with low vision present to rehabilitation professionals. Although the following strategies or approaches are time-proven, some may not work for you nor do all necessarily represent the best approach to solving your individual challenges. Since everyone's vision and personal circumstances are different, there is no substitute for direct consultation with a specialist who has a background in the rehabilitation of people who are blind or have visual impairments.

If you are reading this because your concerns are about a child or an adult of working age, please see Appendix B for a listing of the vocational rehabilitation services in North America. For information about educational services, contact your state's department of public education.

Because this book is distributed throughout North America, as well as overseas, the term "state agency" includes services provided by your province or other comparable unit of government.

❖ Acknowledgments

We would like to thank the following people and organizations for their help in putting this book together: The Wisconsin Council of the Blind, Madison, WI; Dr. Stephen Kessler, Middleton, WI; Eschenbach Optik of America, Ridgefield, CT; TeleSensory, Inc., Mountain View, CA; MaxiAids, Farmingdale, NY; Ocutech, Inc., Chapel Hill, NC; Lighthouse Low Vision Products, Long Island City, NY; Donegan Optical Co., Lenexa, KS; Lynne Luxton, New York, NY; Penne Canterbury, Eau Claire, WI; Betsy True, Madison, WI.

To Lisa, Rebecca, and Elliot — MEF

To the people with low vision who have taught me so much — DJG

To the people who continue to be committed to providing high quality vision rehabilitation services — BLM

Chapter 1

What is Low Vision?

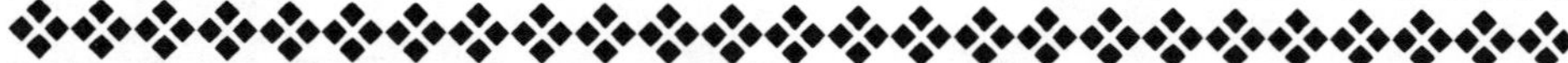

There is much confusion about the various terms used in the field of vision rehabilitation. Probably the most confusing are those that describe the levels of vision and vision impairment. Almost everyone has heard the term "legally blind," but few know exactly what it means. In fact, most people assume it means that a person has no usable vision, but this is not usually the case. Let's begin by considering the range of possibilities on the whole spectrum of vision for humans.

20/20 Vision

Average, or "normal," vision ranges from **20/20** (read as "twenty over twenty" or "twenty-twenty") to 20/40. These are numbers we have all heard at some time in our lives, but what do they mean? In the late 19th century, a Dutch ophthalmologist named Snellen created a chart for measuring visual acuity that used letters of various sizes. Today, the term **20/20** is understood to mean perfect vision, when, in fact, it means average vision. The first or top number in the fraction or ratio indicates the distance of the eye from the eye chart. The standard distance is 20 feet, or 6 meters. The second or bottom number in the fraction or ratio indicates the size of the symbol that was clearly seen. So the visual acuity 20/20 means that the eye could see at 20 feet a symbol (letter, number, or picture) of the size that can be seen by the average eye at 20 feet. The measurement of 20/200 means that at a distance of 20 feet the eye could see a symbol that could be seen by the average eye 200 feet away.

Low Vision

The term **low vision** has no official definition. It is generally considered to be an impairment of vision that limits the things a person wants to do but is not total blindness. Most people with low vision can get around a familiar house or apartment safely and independently and can take care of themselves in most areas of their lives. However, people with low vision will probably have difficulty with reading and writing and handling some common daily living activities, and they may not be able to drive a car.

People with low vision may have a **mild** impairment that prevents them from reading small print. They may find that, with extra light or the use of a hand-held magnifier, it is possible to "get by" in most of their daily activities. Those with a more **severe** impairment will have greater difficulty reading even with a magnifier. They will no longer be able to drive and will be considered to be legally blind. People with an **extensive** loss of vision will require such high amounts of magnification for reading that reading lengthy printed materials will probably be possible for only the most persistent and motivated individuals. People with extensive vision loss may find they need to rely on recorded materials or braille (a raised dot system of reading and writing) for most or much of their reading.

Blindness

Blindness is a word evoking fear and concern in many people. Today, there is some debate about how to define the term and who should and should not be labeled as blind. Originally, the term *blind* included all people with impaired eyesight who could not readily meet society's expectations of sighted abilities. With advances in medicine and improved access to rehabilitation and education, more people with various levels of impaired vision are able to equally participate in the mainstream of modern life. Some people prefer to use the word blind to identify all people with visual impairments. On the other hand, there are those who believe that the word blind should be reserved to identify those with little or no usable vision. The term *low vision* should be used for those people with some usable vision. Some might also suggest that the term *visually impaired* be designated to cover the entire group of people who are blind or have low vision.

Legal Blindness

Most people have a visual acuity of about 20/20 while wearing their glasses or contact lenses (if needed). Those who are **legally blind** have a visual acuity of no better than 20/200 in their better eye with their glasses or contact lenses. It is commonly thought that people in this group have little or no useful vision, but this is usually not the case. In fact, 80–85 percent of all people who are legally blind have some usable vision.

Although many people think that blurry or cloudy vision is the only aspect of visual impairment, there is another way in which loss of function can occur. This is through the loss of peripheral or side vision — the loss of visual field. This is sometimes referred to as "tunnel vision." People are considered legally blind if their central visual field in their better eye is no greater than 20 degrees (normal vision in one eye is about 140 degrees). This is the case regardless of how clear the acuity is. Some legally blind people have 20/20 vision and don't even need glasses! However, they can only see through a small pinhole, or tunnel, of vision. This type of vision loss can also have a great impact on one's ability to function independently. *Legal blindness*, then, is a term used to identify one's status for medical or governmental purposes. It does not necessarily tell us much about how well or how poorly a person sees.

Total Blindness

People who are totally blind or have no useful vision should not be forgotten. Although this book was written to help those with some usable remaining vision, people who are totally blind will probably receive services from many of the same agencies and professionals as people with low vision. In blindness rehabilitation, there is no distinct separation between these two groups. In fact, many people with low vision find it easier to do some activities nonvisually rather than to continue struggling to see through the blur. Also, many people have vision that changes from day to day or from morning to afternoon. If this is the case, it may be beneficial to learn alternative nonvisual techniques. Mainly, it is important to remember that many of the differences between living with limited vision and living with little or no vision can be adequately bridged.

Chapter 2

Who has Low Vision?

Although there have been many recent advances in the treatment of eye conditions, such progress has not kept pace with the unprecedented medical advances enabling people to live longer. In simple terms, the older you are, the more likely you are to develop a visual impairment or become legally blind.

According to the American Foundation for the Blind (Kirchner, 1988), one out of every eight persons in the United States is more than age 65. This represents approximately 30 million people. While the under-65 population increased by 6 percent during the 1980s, those over 65 increased by 17 percent. It is predicted that by the year 2020, the number of people, 85 and older, will be double the population level of 1985.

This "greying of America" trend is creating a large group of older people who are at higher risk of developing low vision. According to the American Foundation for the Blind of New York, approximately two thirds of all people who are severely visually impaired (unable to read newsprint with their best pair of glasses) are 65 or older, more than one-fifth are between 45 and 64, with the remaining 9 percent under 45.

One way to look at this is to say that nearly one out of every six Americans age 65 or older is blind or has a severe visual impairment. Of persons over age 85, one out of every four is severely visually impaired.

As you can see, there is a growing number of people who share the frustrations and challenges of coping with low vision in their later years.

Gender Differences

Gender differences among people with visual impairments become more distinct as the population ages. A large gap exists between the number of males and females, age 65 and older, who are visually impaired.

Women in this older age group represent almost 46 percent of all people with severe visual impairments, while males represent 24 percent (the remaining 30 percent are under age 65). This is not to say that being a woman means you are more likely to have a condition that will cause you to have poor vision. Because a woman's life expectancy in the United States is about 7 years greater than a man's, more women live to the age where visual impairments are quite common. Again, you are more likely to have a visual impairment at 82 than at 72, whether you are a male or a female.

Women in the middle age, 45 to 64, group (almost 13 percent) still outnumber men (9 percent) among those with severe visual impairments, but the distribution is closer.

In the birth-to-44 age range, more males (5.3 percent) than females (4 percent) have severe visual impairments.

Racial Differences

Members of racial or ethnic minorities have a rate of visual impairment 33 percent higher than members of the white population. African-Americans, Hispanics,

Asians/Pacific Islanders, and Native Americans have a rate of about 88 persons with severe visual impairments per 10,000. Caucasians have a rate of 62 per 10,000.

The racial discrepancies may partially result from economic, social, or cultural conditions, but such factors cannot totally explain the differences. African-Americans are much more likely than Caucasians to have glaucoma, and Native Americans are more likely to have diabetes — both of which can lead to vision loss. If you belong to either of these groups, you should have your eye pressure and blood sugar level monitored regularly.

The diagrams on pages 10 and 11 present the age-related trends in blindness and visual impairment.

Blindness Population Estimates

Ages	*Rate per 100,000*	*U.S. Blind Population*
All ages	241	589,700
75 and over	1,860	222,200
65 through 74	637	111,400
45 through 64	146	112,100
20 through 44	106	102,700
5 through 19	62	33,500
Under 5	42	7,800

Severely Visually Impaired Population Estimates

Ages	*Rate per 100,000*	*U.S. Severely Visually Impaired Population*
All ages	1,155	2,823,700
75 and over	13,000	1,552,700
65 through 74	4,700	822,000
45 through 64	600	273,400
18 through 44	130	137,300
Under 18	60	38,300

(Adapted from *Data on Blindness and Visual Impairment in the U.S.*, Second Edition, by Corrine Kirchner, American Foundation for the Blind, New York, NY.)

Chapter 3

The Eye and the Visual System

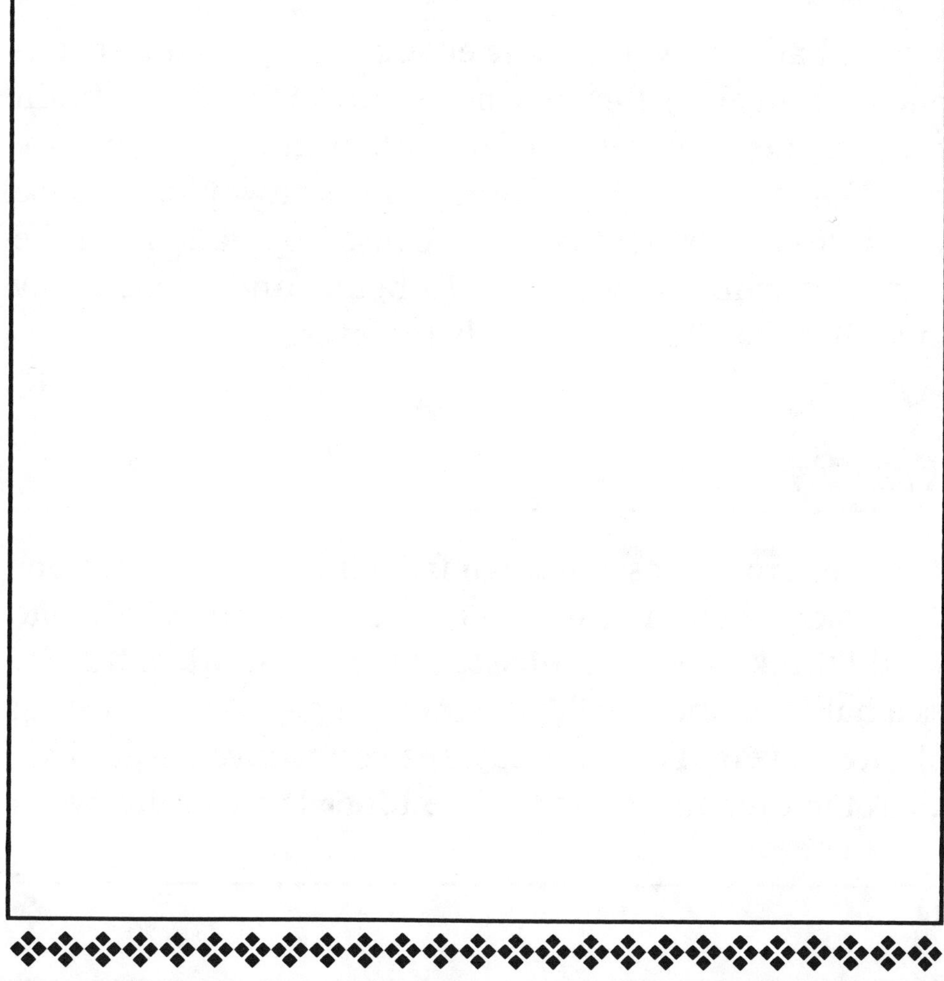

Helping people understand how their eyes work and why they don't work is one of the most important things done as part of vision rehabilitation. It is not necessary for most people to obtain a deep understanding of the structure (anatomy) or the diseases (pathology) of the eye. But most of us grew up learning little about our eyes and have relied on our health care providers to take care of them for us. This chapter discusses in plain language how our eyes work.

The visual system is made up of three basic parts:

1. The eyes
2. The optic nerves
3. The brain

Vision happens when light enters the eyes and an impulse is sent along the optic nerves to the brain. The brain receives the impulses and gives them meaning, and we see. Damage anywhere along the pathway can cause vision loss. Most low vision is caused by damage to the nerve layer inside the eyes. To better understand how this all works, let's start with the eyes.

The Eyes

The eyes are organs, although from the way we commonly speak of them (i.e., stronger, weaker, getting tired), one would think they were muscles. One can think of the eye as a ball or globe (see the diagram on page 15) consisting of three layers. The outer layer is connective tissue. This gives the eyeball its shape. The inner layer of the eye is

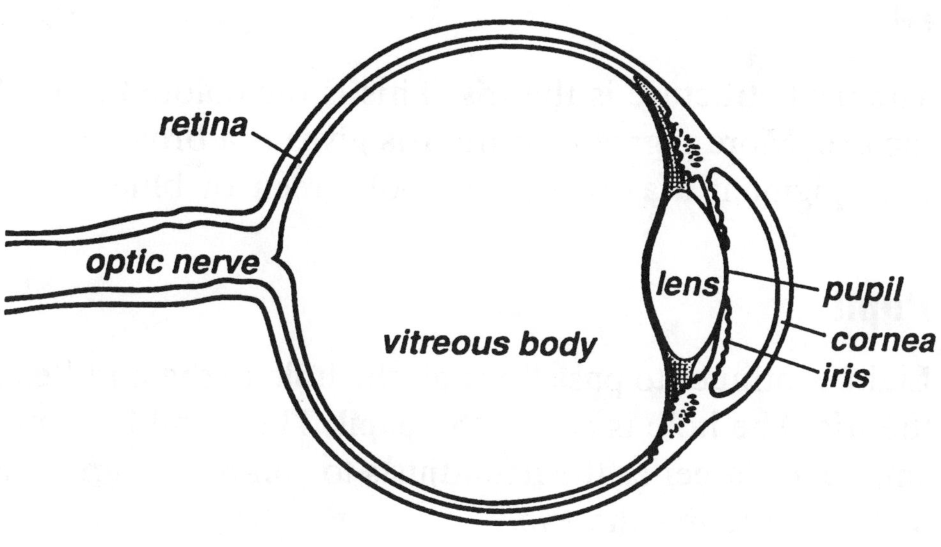

Cross section of the eye.

nerve tissue. It is the same material one's brain is made of and is considered part of the central nervous system. The middle layer is the blood vessel layer that takes nourishment to the nerve layer cells and removes their waste. The large cavity in the middle of the eye, the **vitreous** (vih TREE us) chamber, is filled with a clear, gelatin-like material that also helps to give the eyeball its shape.

Cornea

Light enters through the **cornea** (CORE nee ah), the clear window in the front of the eye. This is the part of the eye that feels pain or irritation when we get dust in our eye. The cornea helps to focus the light rays entering the eye.

Iris

The next structure is the **iris.** This is the colored part of the eye. More pigment in the iris gives it a brown color. Less pigment makes the iris look green or blue.

Pupil

Light continues to pass through the hole in the middle of the iris. The hole is called the **pupil.** The pupil becomes smaller or larger as the iris adjusts to control the amount of light entering the eye.

Lens

Directly behind the pupil sits the eye's own crystalline **lens.** The lens becomes thicker or thinner as you focus close or far away.

Retina, Optic Nerve, and Brain

Light continues to pass through the vitreous chamber until it lands on the inner lining of the eye, the **retina** (REH teh na). At this point, light-sensitive (photoreceptor) cells absorb the light energy and send a message of what has been received through a bundle of nerve fibers called the **optic nerve.** This nerve is connected to the portion of the **brain** that reads and interprets the impulse. The image is recognized by the brain's memory bank and the process of sight is completed.

When any part of this system is damaged, vision will be altered.

Chapter 4

Diseases of the Eye

The major diseases of the eye that affect older people are each listed with a brief, simple description.

Age-Related Maculopathy

Age-related maculopathy (Maa cue LAW paa thee) is the leading cause of vision loss in older Americans. It is also known as macular degeneration, senile macular degeneration, or age-related macular degeneration. It is a disease that affects the blood vessel layer underneath the retina. Changes or damage to these blood vessels cause degeneration of the nerve tissue. The nerve tissue is responsible for receiving the image of what you are trying to see. Only a very small part of the retina is affected. This area is called the **macula.** Although it is only about one-fifth of an inch across, it is the part of the eye that allows one to see the details in things such as print or people's faces. It is also where most of the cells responsible for color vision are concentrated. The center of the macula is called the **fovea** and it is only as big as the period at the end of this sentence. This area is even more sensitive and important for decoding the details of an image.

There are two types of age-related maculopathy. The "dry" type and the "wet" type.

Dry Age-Related Maculopathy

About 90 percent of the cases of age-related maculopathy are the **dry** or **atrophic** type. In this condition, the small blood vessels underneath the macula dry up, and the nerve cells the blood vessels were nourishing slowly degenerate and die. This is perceived as a slow and gradual decrease in vision that initially may be misunderstood as a need for a change in glasses. At present, there is no treatment for this condition.

Wet Age-Related Maculopathy

The second type of age-related maculopathy is called the **wet** or **exudative** type. In this condition, blood vessels under the macula begin to leak or hemorrhage, causing a separation of the layers of cells in the retina. As the blood or blood fluids leak from the vessels, the layers of the retinal cells separate. In some cases, laser surgery can be used to stop the leakage or control the damage from the leakage. Many times, however, the problem is not discovered until it is too late for effective treatment. In some cases, the location of the leak is too close to the fovea to permit treatment. A person with "wet" age-related maculopathy can experience a sudden change in vision and often notices distortions in the vision, such as straight lines that appear to be crooked or wavy.

With age-related maculopathy, a person usually ends up with a **central blind spot** called a **scotoma** (skoh TOME ah). The side, or peripheral, vision is still intact, and you can learn to use this quite efficiently. You will never go completely blind from this condition alone, but you may be severely restricted in such activities as driving or reading the newspaper.

Diabetic Retinopathy

Diabetic retinopathy (RHET in ah pah thee), or the eye disease that may result from long-term diabetes, is another leading cause of vision impairment in older people. This is also a disease that changes the blood vessels that, in turn, causes damage to the nerve layer or retina. Serious vision-threatening complications of diabetic retinopathy occur with a leak or hemorrhage of blood vessels under the retina or of new blood vessels that have grown on top of the retina. In other cases, the retina may become detached from the blood vessel layer underneath it. This is also very serious and may cause a total, permanent loss of vision. Fortunately, early detection and treatment of diabetic eye disease has proved to be very effective in reducing the amount of vision loss and the number of cases of blindness. You may think that only those with diabetes requiring insulin injections are prone to vision complications. Actually, people who take pills for diabetes or control it by diet and exercise may develop vision problems as well. People with diabetes should see their eye care specialist for *dilated* eye exams on a regular basis (based on the advice of the doctor). You should not wait until a change in vision is noticed before making an appointment.

Glaucoma

Glaucoma (glaw COE mah) is the condition in which the pressure of the fluid inside the eye increases to cause damage to the optic nerve in the back of the eye. This damage leads to a gradual decrease in peripheral, or side, vision before affecting central, or straight-ahead, vision. As you are more aware of central vision, it is extremely difficult to detect whether you have glaucoma by how your eyes feel or how you see. Glaucoma is detected and measured by checking the pressure within the eyes, examining the optic nerves, and by measuring the side vision (visual fields). Often, it can be controlled with medication, usually eye drops.

Cataracts

Cataracts (CAA tah rax) occur often with aging. In this condition, the crystalline lens inside the eye becomes cloudy. Cataracts are not a disease or abnormal growth in the eye and in most cases may now be easily and safely removed through surgery. Cataract extraction is the most common surgical procedure in the United States. In the past, people needed to wear thick glasses after cataract surgery to obtain their best vision. Today, most people are able to use the intraocular lens (sometimes called an "I.O.L." or an "implant"). This is a tiny plastic disc implanted in the eye during cataract surgery. It takes the place of the cloudy lens that was removed and permits the person to wear conventional glasses.

Retinal Vascular Occlusions

Retinal vascular occlusions are blockages of arteries or veins in the retina. The amount of vision affected depends on the location and extent of the blockage of the blood vessel. In some cases, your eye doctor may be able to recommend laser surgery to restore vision or prevent further loss of vision. In other cases, your doctor will examine your eyes on a regular basis and let nature take its course.

Hemianopia

A hemianopia (HIM ee aa no pee ah) is one of the visual effects that can occur after a stroke or other injury that affects the supply of blood to the brain. When the part of the brain that reads the signals sent to it by the eye is damaged in a stroke, that part of the visual system is no longer able to process information from the eyes. Sometimes the condition may involve the right side of both eyes or the left side of both eyes. Then it is called a homonymous hemianopia. If the area of the brain responsible for sharp, central vision is not affected, good visual acuity may remain. However, if this particular area is involved, the acuity may be quite low. Even when a person can still see clearly, this type of visual field loss can make such tasks as writing or reading quite difficult.

Chapter 5

Myths About the Eyes

There is a great deal of misunderstanding about the eyes and vision. Some of the more common misunderstandings are discussed here. Of course, it is always best to consult an eye care professional if you have specific questions.

Use of the Eyes

"You can damage your eyes by overusing them."

"Reading in poor light will damage your eyes."

"Reading fine print or doing fine work such as embroidery will damage your eyes."

"Sitting too close to the TV will damage your eyes."

"Flashes of bright light, for example, flash photography, will damage your eyes."

It is important that older people, especially those with visual impairments, understand and believe that they cannot damage or "use up" vision by using existing eyesight. Although an individual may experience discomfort performing a task, such as reading, for an extended period of time or by struggling to accomplish a similar activity in low levels of light, he or she is not damaging the eye. However, you may experience mental fatigue or strain to the external eye muscles that control the movements of the eye. This does not lead to any eyesight impairment. Most people should be encouraged to use their remaining vision as much as possible.

Glasses

"Glasses make your eyes stronger."

"Not wearing glasses makes your eyes weaker."

"If you wear glasses, your eyes will become dependent on them and become weaker."

"Wearing someone else's glasses will ruin your eyes."

"Glass lenses are better than plastic lenses."

Glasses are simply tools that help the eye to focus light on the nerve layer, or retina. They can help you to use your eyes comfortably and efficiently but do not affect the health of the eye. Wearing glasses will not make your eyes weaker, stronger, or dependent on glasses. Wearing someone else's glasses may give you a headache, but it will not hurt your eyes. You can wear either glass or plastic lenses, they both do the same job equally well.

Medical Myths

"Carrots make your eyesight better."

"Vitamins and minerals will improve eyesight or prevent eye disease."

"The eye can be transplanted."

"During eye surgery, the eye is removed and then replaced."

"A person can get AIDS through contact with contaminated tears."

The body requires a variety of vitamins and minerals to maintain good health, and Vitamin A is important in the development and maintenance of good vision. Consumption of amounts beyond the minimum adult daily requirement of Vitamin A or foods rich in Vitamin A, such as carrots, will not produce stronger vision. The use of vitamin and mineral supplements, such as zinc, to prevent eye disease in older people is under study at this time. Remember that excessive amounts of virtually any substance can be detrimental to one's health. Vitamin A and zinc can be toxic in large amounts.

One of the most common myths about eye surgery is that the eye can be removed and replaced, and, therefore, it is possible to transplant the eye. It is true that the eye can be removed, but it cannot be reattached to the optic nerve. Transplantation of the cornea is often misunderstood as transplantation of the whole eye. Also, the terms "transplant" and "implant" (the intraocular lens implant that is usually a part of cataract surgery) are often confused.

There is no record of any person contracting AIDS through tears or from exchanging contact lenses. However, like all body fluids, tears can contain the virus that causes AIDS.

Because the eyes and the visual system are so complex, it is not surprising that there are so many misunderstandings about them. Most people have not had the opportunity or the need to learn about their eyes to prepare them for coping with vision loss. If you have further questions about your eyes, ask your eye doctor and his or her staff.

Chapter 6

Care of the Eyes

Prevention of Vision Loss

Although older people as a group are most likely to need professional eye care, they may also be the group least likely to identify abnormal changes and seek help for a number of complex and interrelated reasons. First, an older person may consider vision decline a normal part of the aging process. Although a reduction in near vision and night vision will occur with aging, it should no longer be considered the rule that older people will become severely visually impaired. In fact, most older people in the United States do not experience serious age-related vision impairments.

Second, older people may have grown up in a social environment that encouraged such complete trust in doctors that they may assume any abnormality in their vision is acceptable unless their doctor has told them differently. Most people do not routinely test their vision in a standardized way and one eye at a time. This makes it difficult for the average person to notice if the vision has changed in one eye but not in the other.

Amsler Grid

The Amsler grid test is a very important and simple method of assessing certain eye problems at an early stage, when treatment might be beneficial. The test consists of a black and white grid of small squares on a sheet of paper (see page 29; additional copies are available from your eye doctor). You look at the grid to detect distortions or the loss of areas of central vision. This is a very

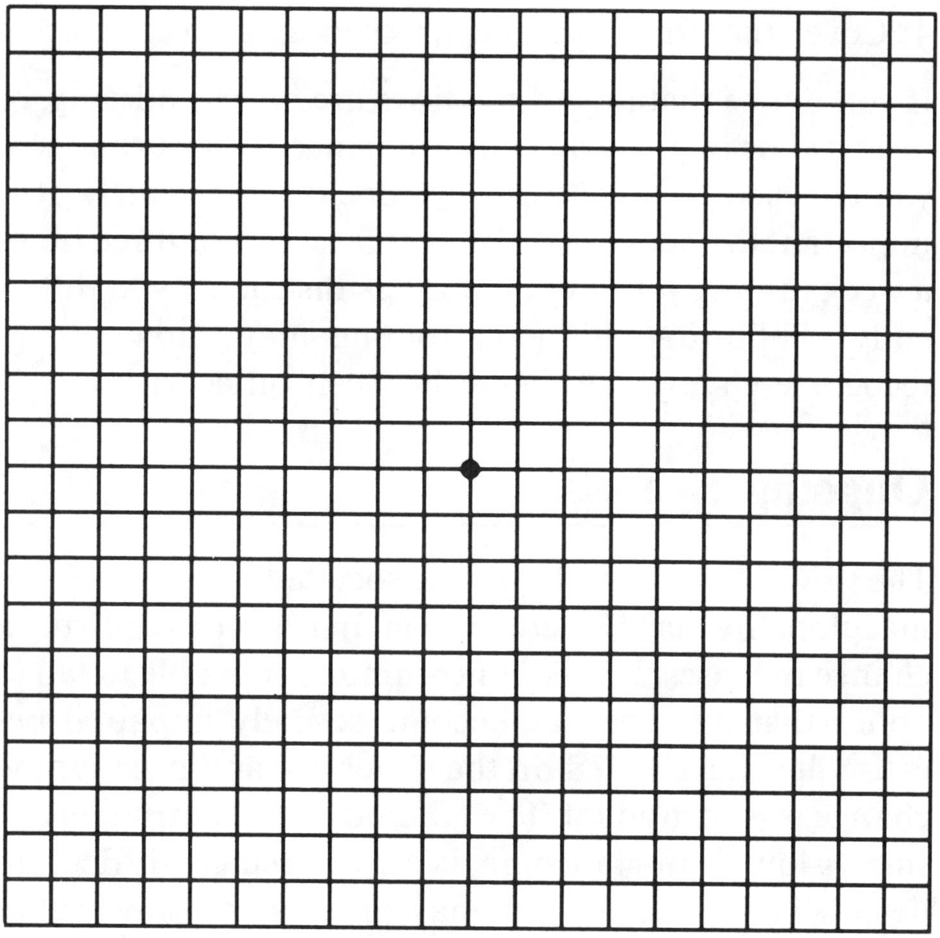

The Amsler grid test

easy test to do at home and can help in the early detection or the progression of macular degeneration.

1. Hold the grid in your hand or tape it on the bathroom mirror, medicine cabinet, or wall.
2. Place the grid at arm's length.
3. Cover one eye, look at the spot in the center of the grid. Do not move your eyes or look at the other areas of the grid. Are the horizontal or vertical lines distorted?

4. Cover the other eye and proceed as above.

If you notice that any of the lines are blurry, missing, or distorted or in any way changed (since the last time that you checked), contact your eye doctor **immediately**. It is important to check your vision at least two or three times a week (unless your eye doctor has instructed you differently). Following this easy routine may allow you to recognize changes in vision between office visits.

Ongoing Eye Care

The slow loss of central vision associated with age-related maculopathy may be perceived at first as only requiring a change in lenses. It is not uncommon for people to fail to notice that one eye has become severely impaired because they have relied on the better eye and because the change was so gradual. The gradual loss of peripheral, or side vision, as in glaucoma, is also extremely difficult to detect. This is because it may progress so slowly that changes can only be noted from year to year. Nevertheless, permanent and irreversible damage is being done.

Often a person with one severe eye problem, such as age-related maculopathy, will be told that "nothing more can be done." Older people might mistake this statement as meaning that there is no need for an eye care professional to monitor the health of the eyes, and they may simply stop going to the eye doctor. After all, people go to the doctor with the expectation that "something" will be done.

Older people should see an eye care specialist at least every other year if not recommended more often by their eye doctor. The appointment should include an examination in which eye drops are used to enlarge your pupils (a dilated examination) and a measure of the pressure inside your eyes (glaucoma test).

Safety Glasses

People who have useful vision in only one eye should be encouraged to talk to their eye care professional about the value of wearing protective lenses (safety glasses) during their waking hours. This protective measure is often overlooked, especially with older people who may not be engaged in an active lifestyle. However, as many people are wearing glasses anyway, making the lens out of a safety material, such as polycarbonate (a high-strength, nearly unbreakable plastic), is only slightly more expensive and provides greater protection.

Health Maintenance

If you already have low vision, you should not risk losing useful vision because of an undiagnosed condition. General care of the eyes through regular examinations not only establishes your current visual ability, but also helps in the early detection of diseases. Early detection and timely treatment can often help maintain usable remaining vision.

Glaucoma, for example, can usually be successfully treated with eye drops if detected early. Glaucoma has been referred to as the "sneak thief of sight" because it is usually painless and develops gradually. Although treatment will not improve your vision, it will prevent further loss.

Age-related maculopathy, cataracts, glaucoma, and diabetic and vascular retinopathies, as discussed previously, are diseases that can lead to a major loss of vision if not detected early and treated properly. Therefore, a complete eye examination will include tests for each of these.

The National Society to Prevent Blindness suggests that people over 40 have their eyes checked by an eye care specialist at least once every other year. If you have diabetes or glaucoma, there is a need for more frequent appointments. You should discuss the need and frequency for a regular eye health examination with your doctor.

Vision Screening

Vision screening, offered at work, a senior citizen center, or health fair, is only done to identify whether you are at risk for a vision loss. A screening is usually limited to a measure of the pressure inside your eyes (glaucoma test), but can sometimes include testing for how clearly you can see (visual acuity). A test for how much area you can see (visual field test) may also be done.

A screening is not a complete vision evaluation. A "normal" finding does not assure that the eyes are healthy and without disease. If a problem is detected, a complete exam by an eye doctor is the most appropriate way to find out more about it. Remember, early detection and treatment should help maintain the eyesight you have. Even if you have a stable eye condition and "nothing more can be done" about it, regular checkups can prevent or detect other problems.

Chapter 7

Eye Care Providers

There are a variety of eye care professionals you may hear about or see. The services they provide may vary, depending on your state's licensing regulations. Because of this, descriptions are general.

Ophthalmologists

Ophthalmologists (awp thawl MAW low jists) are doctors of medicine (M.D.) or osteopathy (D.O.). They are licensed to practice surgery and medicine and can prescribe contact lenses, glasses, and medications. They specialize in all aspects of eye and vision care.

Optometrists

Optometrists are doctors of optometry (O.D.). They are licensed to practice in select areas of eye and vision care. They can evaluate people for visual problems and prescribe glasses or contact lenses. In some states they may use medications to help diagnose and treat diseases.

Opticians

Opticians are technicians who fit, adjust, and sell contact lenses, glasses, protective eyewear, and other optical devices.

Low Vision Therapists

Low vision therapists work with people with impaired vision to help them learn to use special skills and aids to make the best use of their remaining vision.

Others

Ophthalmic nurses are licensed professionals who specialize in care of the eyes.

Ophthalmic assistants, technicians, and technologists are medical assistants who are specially trained to assist the ophthalmologist by collecting information and performing tests.

Orthoptists work with the ophthalmologist and specialize in assessing and treating problems involving the eye muscles or coordination of the two eyes.

Ocularists are specialists in making artificial eyes. They design a cosmetic shell painted to match the original or remaining eye.

Each provider has special services to offer. If you are attempting to cope with impaired vision that cannot be corrected by conventional lenses, surgery, or medicine, you will want to see professionals who work with people with low vision. Rehabilitation specialists are listed in Chapter 11.

Chapter 8

Your Eye Exam

Probably the most important thing you can do for your eyes is to have them examined regularly by an eye doctor. The exam itself actually requires many tests in a brief amount of time. This chapter will help you understand what goes on during your appointment.

When you make your appointment, be prepared to ask the following questions.

Questions to Ask the Office Personnel

Before you see the doctor, ask the office staff the following questions.

1. What will the examination include?
2. If dilating medications are used, will I be able to drive home after the exam?
3. Does the doctor accept all types of insurance?
4. Does the doctor take Medicare assignment?
5. What is the estimated cost of the office visit and the doctor's services?
6. How much money might I expect to need on the day of the appointment for uncovered doctor's services or anticipated prescriptions?
7. Can payment plans be arranged, if necessary?

Costs vary greatly for regular eye examinations, follow-up care for eye conditions, medications, rehabilitation services, special procedures, and/or corrective lenses. If the expense will cause a hardship, ask if there is a social worker or financial counselor available to help you.

Questions to Ask the Insurance Company

You may want to call your insurance provider before the visit and ask the following questions.

1. What portion of the cost of a regular eye examination is covered?
2. Are medications covered, and is a co-payment required?
3. Are any special treatments or procedures covered?
4. Is there an annual limit to my coverage?
5. How can I get specific coverage details in writing?
6. What other services, such as rehabilitation or referrals to other specialists, will my policy cover?

Asking these questions can help you anticipate the cost so you can budget accordingly. If the expense will cause a hardship, ask for information on sources of financial assistance.

Questions to Ask the Eye Doctor

During your appointment you should be prepared to ask the doctor the following questions. It is often helpful to have them written down ahead of time. You may even want to bring this book with you to the examination.

1. What is the name of the eye disease?

2. What caused it?
3. Will it get worse, get better, or stay the same?
4. What can be done about it?
5. Can I do anything to improve or worsen my condition?
6. What follow-up care is needed?
7. Are medications needed?
8. Are my relatives also at risk for developing this condition?
9. Will glasses or new lenses help?
10. What rehabilitation services are available that might benefit me?

Vision Evaluation

A complete vision evaluation includes a health and medication history and several tests. Information about your overall health (including that of your immediate family) and the medications you use will help the doctor determine what tests to perform and how to interpret the findings. The tests are aimed at discovering the workings of different parts of the eye.

History of Your Vision, Health, and Medication Use

For your appointment, you should be able to describe how well you can see and any recent changes in your vision, as well as any problems you've noticed. Make special note (write it down if necessary) of any double or blurry vision, flashes of light, poor night vision, or difficulty focusing, for example.

You will be asked about any health problems you have and the medications you take. Also, you will be asked about your family's general health history. The doctor will want to know about any health problems of your blood relatives.

Be prepared to talk about the following:

1. High blood pressure (hypertension)
2. Eye diseases, such as glaucoma or age-related maculopathy (see Chapter 4)
3. High blood sugar (diabetes)
4. Medications (both prescriptions and over-the-counter)
5. Any injuries or surgeries to the eyes

Visual Acuity Test

The visual acuity test is the testing of both eyes for near and distance vision. It tells how clearly you can see the symbols on the eye chart. This information will help your doctor to determine if you need a change in your glasses.

Refraction

Testing your vision with different lenses to determine if your vision can be improved with glasses or contact lenses is called a refraction. You will be asked to choose between different lenses and to tell the doctor which ones make things clearer.

Intraocular Pressure Test

This test is done to determine the pressure of the fluid within your eyes. The test may be done with either a gentle puff of air or by the use of an instrument called an applanation tonometer. In the latter case, the instrument actually touches the eye. If an applanation tonometer is used, the eye is first numbed with eye drops.

Visual Field Testing

This test is used to determine side, or peripheral, vision. This tells your doctor how much area you can see, not necessarily how well you can see. Your central visual field may be tested with the Amsler grid. (see Chapter 6, page 29).

Color Vision

You will be given a test to determine how well you can see colors. The test may be on a chart with different colored dots and figures.

Dilated Examination

The dilated examination allows observation of the inner structures of the eye. Drops are used to dilate or open the pupil, allowing the doctor to see inside the eye.

Preparing for your exam helps both you and your eye doctor get the most from your appointment. Asking questions of the office personnel and insurance company will clarify the cost, coverage, and payment options. In a similar way, asking questions of the eye doctor will make clear what the eye problem is, the cause, and what can be done about it.

Everyone benefits from asking questions and being prepared.

Chapter 9

Your Feelings About Losing Vision

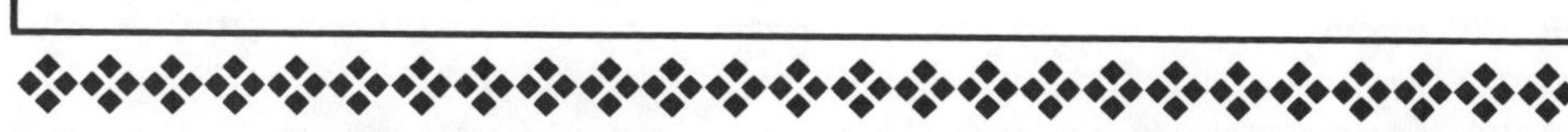

Coping With Your Feelings

Losing vision will affect your feelings in many ways. Your emotional reaction to having low vision will occur:

- When you first learn of your condition, and
- As you meet the challenges of day-to-day living.

The loss of vision will affect how you feel about yourself, the way that you interact with those around you, and how you conduct your daily activities. Your emotional response to the loss of vision is, in large part, determined by your basic personality and how you have adjusted to previous situations or life experiences.

Getting the News

For most people, the first shock comes in their doctor's office. That's where they learn that the blurry vision they have been experiencing is permanent. Many describe the feeling as a "kick in the teeth" or a numbness. How can it be, they may wonder, in a country with such advanced medical technology that there isn't a cure? This is so hard to believe that often people simply don't accept it.

Denial

The difficulty that you may have in accepting your doctor's pronouncement is a typical human response to being told disturbing news. You may say to yourself, "This can't be true. I'll get another opinion. Surely there is someone, somewhere who can treat this condition." Some people point out that no other person in their family has any eye problems, therefore they should not be having this problem. Others believe that if they don't talk about the situation or do anything about the condition, it will go away. All of these responses are different forms of denying what is really happening. Denial is often, although not always, the first way your mind tries to cope with this disturbing new information.

Anger

Another response that you may have to the news of your vision loss is to become angry. Some people get angry at their doctor or an office staff member. Such a patient starts to see everything that person is doing as wrong, careless, or an example of incompetence.

Most people will have some conflicts with those closest to them: a spouse, children, and/or siblings. This can be extremely difficult for everyone involved. People who have just lost their vision may need extra assistance in some areas of their lives, but will not feel comfortable being dependent so much of the time. Family members will want to help relieve the frustration that they see, but may find that they tire of being depended on. Then, they may feel guilty for feeling anything other than a saintly patience. In a similar way, people with vision loss will simultaneously feel gratitude for the extra help and attention they are receiving, but also feel resentment for needing so much help.

Depression

With any loss, including that of losing vision, you may experience a feeling of grief. Grief is a common cause of depression. Some of the signs of depression are isolating one's self from people and activities, losing interest in hobbies, personal neglect, and changes in appetite or sleeping patterns. Other signs of depression include sadness, fatigue, agitation, or loss of interest in life.

Sometimes the sadness may be so great that adjustment to the loss cannot happen. Feelings of being less of a person than before, or that you have less reason to live, cloud your ability to meet the challenges of day-to-day living.

Some people mistakenly believe that a cure for depression is to "cheer up" or to "stop feeling sorry for yourself." However, it is now known that it usually takes more than this to help a person overcome depression. A person who thinks that he or she may be depressed should first talk to their doctor. The doctor should talk to you or arrange for you to talk to a social worker, psychologist, psychiatrist, or some other person who specializes in working with people who may be depressed. The doctor may order some tests to ensure that the depression is not caused by some other physical condition.

Isolation

Because low vision will restrict your ability to drive a car, use public transportation, or even walk independently, it is understandable for you to feel more isolated than at any previous time in your life. For those who are used to getting into their car and driving wherever they wish, this obvious restriction is perhaps the biggest loss experienced with low vision. What may not be quite as apparent are some of the other factors isolating people with low vision.

Because eye conditions are more common among people who are older, members of this group are more likely to have lost some of their close friends to death, be a widow or widower, or have adult children living and working in distant communities. Without having travel companions readily available, you will feel much more limited in your choices of activities or in the times you are able to travel.

Besides being isolated by mobility limitations, you may also experience a different kind of isolation. This is isolation from friends, family, and activities. Some call this "social isolation."

If you are concerned about how you appear to others (Is my clothing neat? Do my socks match? Is my makeup on properly?), you may be less willing to socialize for fear that you will be embarrassed.

When you meet others in public places — people you have known for years — and you can't tell who they are, you may feel very uncomfortable. Others may sense your anxiety or discomfort and be hesitant to interact. If they know of your vision impairment, they may be uncomfortable with that, too. All of this may lead you to think that it just isn't worth going out. This type of isolation builds on itself: The less you go out and do things socially, the less you are motivated to go out.

Acceptance

The final step with learning to live with vision loss is acceptance. Acceptance means coming to terms with the reality of permanent loss. This does not mean that it's easy or occurs overnight. Learning to live with a vision loss is an ongoing process. The process is not always in a forward direction or in a neat series of steps. People frequently reach a point in the adjustment process where they stay for some period of time. Time, experience, physical, psychological, social, and environmental factors encourage movement to the next step.

Learning to live with the vision loss may not be easy. It frequently seems like a fight. Some battles are won and some lost. Some days are good and filled with hope. Other days are bad and filled with frustration. There can be ongoing feelings of frustration and wanting to give up. However, these reactions are not as overwhelming as the initial shock and won't last as long.

A point will come when you adjust to the loss. Adjustment may be experienced in terms of your ability to carry out "normal" activities as independently as possible and also to achieve a realistic perception of the loss. You can use a task, such as cooking, as a standard to judge your progress in adjusting. Looking back, you can see how much has been learned and accomplished. (See Chapter 17 on ways to cope with common daily challenges.)

For many, the adjustment process can be best summarized by this older person's thoughts:

It's something you need to accept, but it's a handicap. To be honest, I would have preferred an arm or a leg over my eyes, but what can you do about it? You have to accept it, but it's definitely a handicap.

Once you've accepted the loss, you need to decide to learn to live with it by dealing with the loss to the best of your ability. You can adapt your habitual way of doing things or learn new ways to accomplish day-to-day tasks. You will never be able to do some things again on your own or in the same way. The focus will change from what you cannot do to what you can do.

Chapter 10

Hallucinations

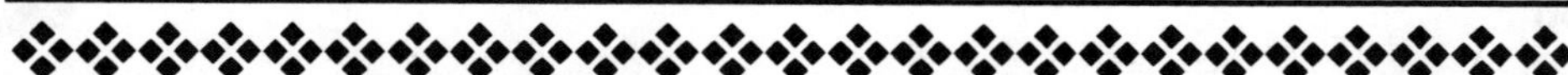

Having visual hallucinations is seeing things that do not exist. This chapter reviews some of the types of visual hallucinations that may be experienced by people with low vision.

Seeing "Shapes"

Many people with low vision, especially those with maculopathy or diabetic retinopathy, notice that they sometimes see shapes, outlines, or pictures in places where they know the things don't really exist. It is common for people to tell rehabilitation professionals that they can see a dark shape in their vision and remark that it looks like something familiar. The shape might remind them of the outline of an animal or the map outline of a state or country. Such images may be noticed most often when first waking up in the morning.

"Patterns"

Other people report that they see patterns in their vision. These have been described as like "looking through broken glass," or that everything has a paisley or flower-like pattern on it. Although these images and distortions can be annoying and even cause concern in some people, most of the time you simply learn to put up with them. This is true for people who have seen their eye doctor and have been assured that these patterns do not require medical treatment.

Distressing Images

Unfortunately, the images and distortions observed by some people are disturbing and frightening. Observing others with apparently misshapen or distorted faces, perceiving patterns of images that look like moving insects, or having the interplay of shadow and light outside their window look like strangers hiding behind a tree or a car can be very disturbing.

What Are They?

There has been little research about the causes of these hallucinations. Probably the phenomenon results from a combination of memory and the eye disease. Perhaps hallucinations are noticed more often in the morning because one is waking up and looking at a blank, light-colored ceiling in the bedroom. Also, the mind may be less cluttered with thoughts and perceptions about the day's activities and may be more apt to notice the outlines, shapes, or patterns in the morning. For people with diabetic eye disease, a hallucination may be caused by the settling of blood cells or the presence of scar tissue.

Perhaps the most negative aspect of hallucinations is the mental and emotional anguish some people go through. They wonder, "Am I losing my mind?" and "If I tell anyone, will they think I'm losing my mind?". Because so many people with low vision have this experience, a low vision support group is probably a safe place to discuss the subject. Undoubtedly, someone else will have had a similar experience. A lot of comfort and reassurance can be gained by knowing that someone else shares your experience and that you are not alone.

Need for Medical Attention

There are some types of visual hallucinations or distortions that could indicate the need for **immediate** medical attention:

1. **Flashing lights** — like firecrackers inside the eye or a dark veil falling on the vision or the sudden appearance of cobwebs — could indicate a torn or detaching retina.
2. **Sudden onset of distortion** — straight lines that look wavy or crooked, like the mirrors in the carnival "fun house" — could indicate age-related maculopathy.
3. **Any sudden change in vision** — requires that you contact your eye doctor immediately and tell him or her exactly what you've noticed.

Although little is known about the distortions and patterns experienced by some people with low vision, it is safe to say that it is a common occurrence. If you have experienced this and are troubled by it, you will probably be helped by talking to someone who understands. Such a person can be found in a support group, a low vision center, or your doctor's office.

Chapter 11

Vision Rehabilitation Services

Vision Rehabilitation

Vision rehabilitation is a service providing people who have low vision with help in getting the most out of their remaining vision. This service is most advantageous when professionals from different disciplines are involved and when the program includes training and education. One "yardstick" you, the consumer, can use to compare different providers is to check to see if:

1. There is an **interdisciplinary** approach.
2. **Training and education** are an important part of the program.

The Interdisciplinary Approach

The interdisciplinary approach means that specialists in different professions work together to help people get the most out of their remaining vision. For example, a model program would include:

- An **eye doctor** making sure that the eyes require no further treatment and that the current eye glasses or contact lenses are the best possible.
- A **low vision therapist** teaching people to use their remaining vision in a more effective way and the efficient use of optical aids.
- A **rehabilitation teacher** providing instruction in activities of daily living and offering information about community resources.

- An **orientation and mobility instructor** teaching independent travel skills and strategies, as well as the use of distance optical aids.
- A **social worker** providing counseling for anger about the loss of vision, or making referrals to other service providers who can help.

In this model program, these specialists may all work under one roof or they may work in separate offices and be several miles apart. Nevertheless, they will be working together or consulting with each other to provide the most complete service possible.

Although you may not need to work with all of the staff listed above, it is important that each staff member have the opportunity to evaluate an individual's needs to determine which services are needed.

Training and Education

Whereas some people can quickly grasp new ideas and methods for using their vision, most can benefit from instruction in the actual use of the aids as well as in how to use their remaining vision. The loaning of trial aids is essential to allow people enough time for practice in their homes or other places the aids will be used. Not only are some new skills being learned, some old ones are being unlearned!

Providing easily understood information about the eyes, the disease(s) that caused the vision loss, and how magnifiers work is an important part of the vision rehabilitation process. Sometimes, these explanations are the most important part of the program. To make informed choices about the types of low vision aids that will be most helpful, people need to have facts and information.

Regardless of how well their eye doctor has explained their eye disease to them, some people can't remember some of the information because of their anxiety. The vision rehabilitation team can review this information and help them understand what is happening. Such questions as: "Will I become completely blind?" or "What did I do to cause this?" can also be answered.

Low Vision Services

Because the most obvious and immediate limitation noticed by people with low vision is their difficulty or inability to read, most people begin their rehabilitation program by looking for "stronger glasses" or a magnifier. If not immediately referred to a vision rehabilitation center, one or more of the following might occur.

The "Wild Goose" Chase

When looking for stronger glasses, people are often told that a more powerful prescription will not help and that a change in their present lenses will make no difference. This doesn't make much sense because, in the past, stronger glasses always helped with reading. If they do find a doctor who will write a new prescription, they are often disappointed because the new glasses aren't much, or any, better than the old ones. They still can't really read well and, in fact, sometimes the old glasses seem better.

Another common occurrence is when a magnifier is purchased at a hobby shop or drug store, or when an old one that has been in the family for years is retrieved from its resting place. Although these sometimes work, many people find these to be only a little bit helpful. If the magnifier they locate has a little "bifocal" or small spot of higher magnification about the size of a dime, they will struggle to read using this small area, as it is the best they can find.

Some people persist and learn about someone who has some stronger lenses. When they meet with this person they are shown a magnifier. If the first one doesn't work, a stronger one is tried. If this is unsuccessful, a yet stronger one is evaluated until the "strongest" has been tried. Although the print is readable, only a few letters or words at a time can be seen.

Equally distressing is the encounter some have with the specialist who writes a prescription for a stronger lens or magnifier, but doesn't provide training in how to use it, doesn't have any loaners available for home trial, and doesn't follow up to see how the aid is working.

With all these obstacles, it's not surprising that many people give up in their search for professional help.

Quality Low Vision Services

Low vision services are provided in different ways by different providers, and there is no single "right" method.

This could be said of many other activities, from home repair to cooking. Each person who does a job will do it a little bit differently, based on the way that he or she has been trained and one's own personal style.

There are currently no national standards for low vision providers, and there is only one agency that certifies low vision centers. This is the National Accreditation Council for Agencies Serving the Blind and Visually Impaired, or NAC (see Appendix A). Some states do have standards or guidelines for providers, and you can check with your state's services for the blind (see Appendix B) to learn about the standards for your area.

Although it is not possible to describe the specifics of a quality low vision clinic, in general, the interdisciplinary approach and an emphasis on training and education as described previously should be present. The availability of low vision aids for loan is also an important feature of quality low vision care. The best interests of the person with low vision should be at the heart of the program, with the evaluation and recommendations based on his or her needs. This may seem obvious, but it is worth investigating.

Questions to Ask the Vision Rehabilitation Provider

1. What disciplines are represented by the staff who will be working with me?

2. Is training in the use of low vision aids and/or remaining vision provided? If so, by whom?

3. What will be covered in the appointment? How long will it take?
4. How much will the service cost? Is this covered by insurance? Are there any other sources of financial assistance available?
5. Are follow-up visits provided? Is the cost for these included in the initial fee?
6. Are aids available for loan? Is there any extra charge for this?

Differing Needs

If your goal is to read newsprint, then the low vision professional should show you if, and how, that can be done. If your goal is to read large print, then it may not be in your best interest to finish the evaluation with a magnifier that is best for newsprint. Most people seek out a low vision provider because they want to "see better." The job of the specialist is to gather information about the client's needs and goals and cooperatively develop a plan to meet them.

For example, two 70-year-old people with age-related maculopathy who have the same visual acuity might have very different goals and seek different solutions for their situations. If one is a retired stock broker who actively manages her own portfolio, she will need to be able to read the stock market section in the newspaper. If the other is a person who did little reading previously, the ability to read a large-print monthly magazine might be his number one goal. These two people with similar situations would have very different magnification needs. The low vision professional you work with should understand such differences in individual needs.

For most people with low vision, obtaining useful services is more involved than simply picking out a magnifier or a "stronger lens." It is worth the time and effort to look into the type of service you will be receiving before you make the appointment.

Chapter 12

Optical Aids

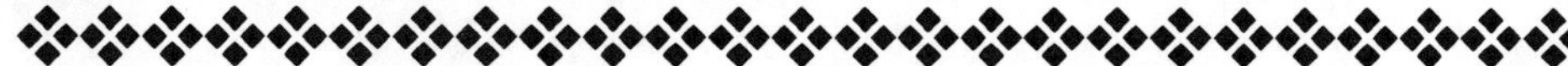

Optical Aids

The task of selecting a low vision aid or aids can be confusing and frustrating. There are often many choices of styles and manufacturers. Most people who have low vision know little about how these devices work or how to use them properly. This chapter describes some of the basic devices you should be familiar with.

Lenses

Until the last 10 to 15 years, optical aids for people with low vision were mostly hand-held magnifiers manufactured for people with average vision who were engaged in a hobby such as stamp or coin collecting. Fortunately, a lot has changed, and people with low vision can now choose from a wide variety of optical aids in different styles from competing companies. Although it is not necessary to know the optics of the various designs, it is important that a magnifying lens be of high quality and that it is designed for people with low vision.

The lenses of the magnifiers designed for people with low vision will provide a clear image all the way to the edge of the lens. Perhaps you remember using an old magnifying glass that magnified clearly in the center but left the rest of the image distorted. These will not work well as low vision aids.

Selecting a Low Vision Aid

Selecting an optical aid requires the consideration of many factors.

1. How will the aid be used?
2. How much magnification is required for the task(s)?
3. What is the physical and emotional condition of the user?
4. Is cost an issue?

Every low vision aid has its own positive and negative features. Some of these features may be positive for one person and negative for another. The low vision therapist should help you sort out these pros and cons but, in the end, you will have to decide which one(s) works best for you.

What follows is a list of the different types of low vision aids and some of the features of each type.

Hand-held Magnifiers

Hand-held magnifiers, like those shown on the next page, are familiar to most people and are generally easy to use. They tend to be inexpensive and can be used at a "normal" working distance (the distance from the eye to the material being viewed). However, hand-held magnifiers must be held steadily and at an exact distance from

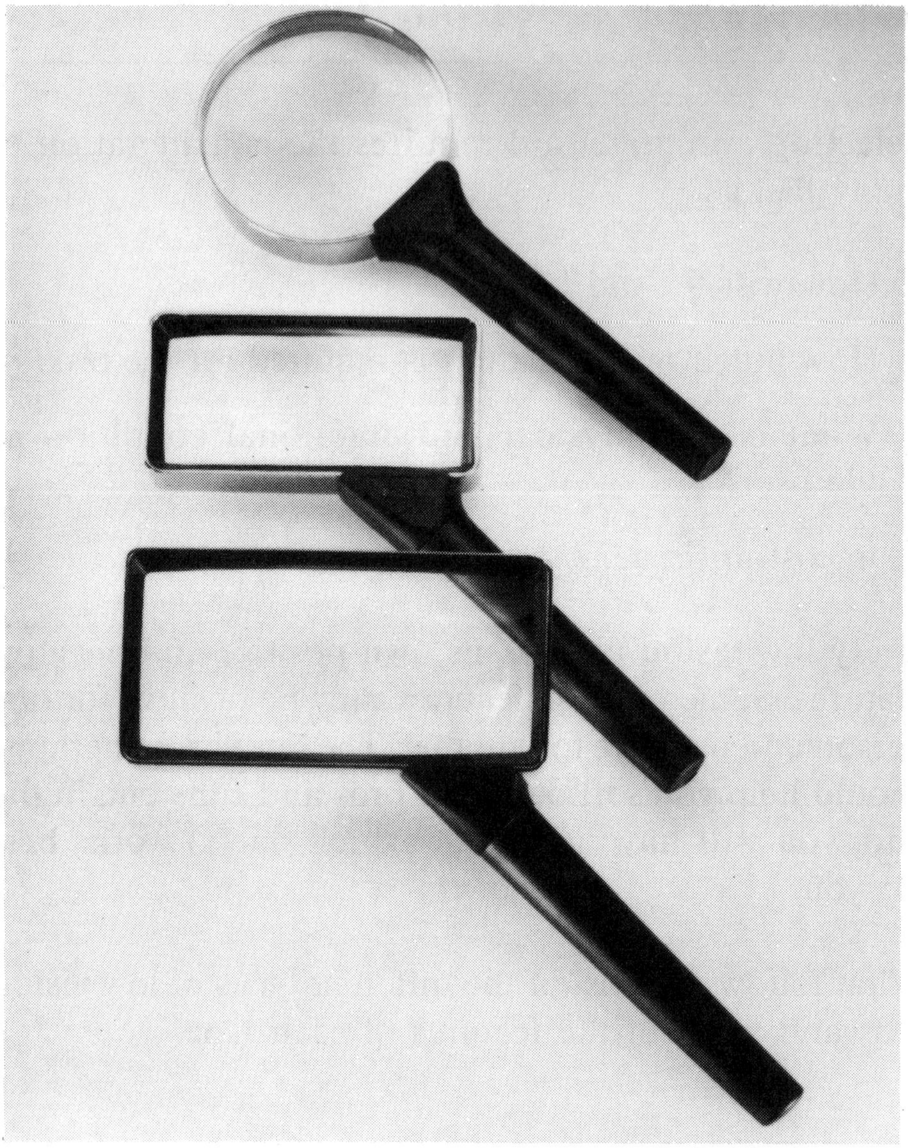

Photo courtesy of Maxi-Aids

Hand-held magnifier.

the print to obtain the maximum amount of magnification. One hand is always tied up holding the magnifier. The area that can be seen will be limited to the size of the magnifier frame, and this may slow reading.

Stand Magnifiers

A stand magnifier, shown on the next page, is like a hand-held magnifier except for the addition of legs or a base to hold the lens steadily at the proper distance from the page. This also means that the focus cannot be changed by moving it closer or farther from the page. There are a few magnifiers with folding supports that can be either hand-held or stand style. You must wear your reading glasses or bifocals to obtain the best focus. Otherwise, it has the same positive and negative features as a hand-held magnifier.

Illuminated Magnifiers

Some magnifiers, like those shown on page 73, have built-in lights and are called illuminated magnifiers. These can be either the hand-held or stand style. The source of power for the light can be either household current (AC), regular batteries, or rechargeable batteries. There is even a choice of the type of bulb, which can be regular incandescent, halogen, or fluorescent.

Most of the time, the presence of extra light when using a magnifier for reading is a positive feature. Your own needs and your intended use for the magnifier will help determine which type is best for you. For example, if the magnifier is to be used primarily in one place, such as your favorite chair, it probably makes sense to use one with a plug-in power source for the light. A battery-powered light is more suitable for short-term reading and is much more portable. The type of light is a personal choice, with each person having his or her likes and dis-

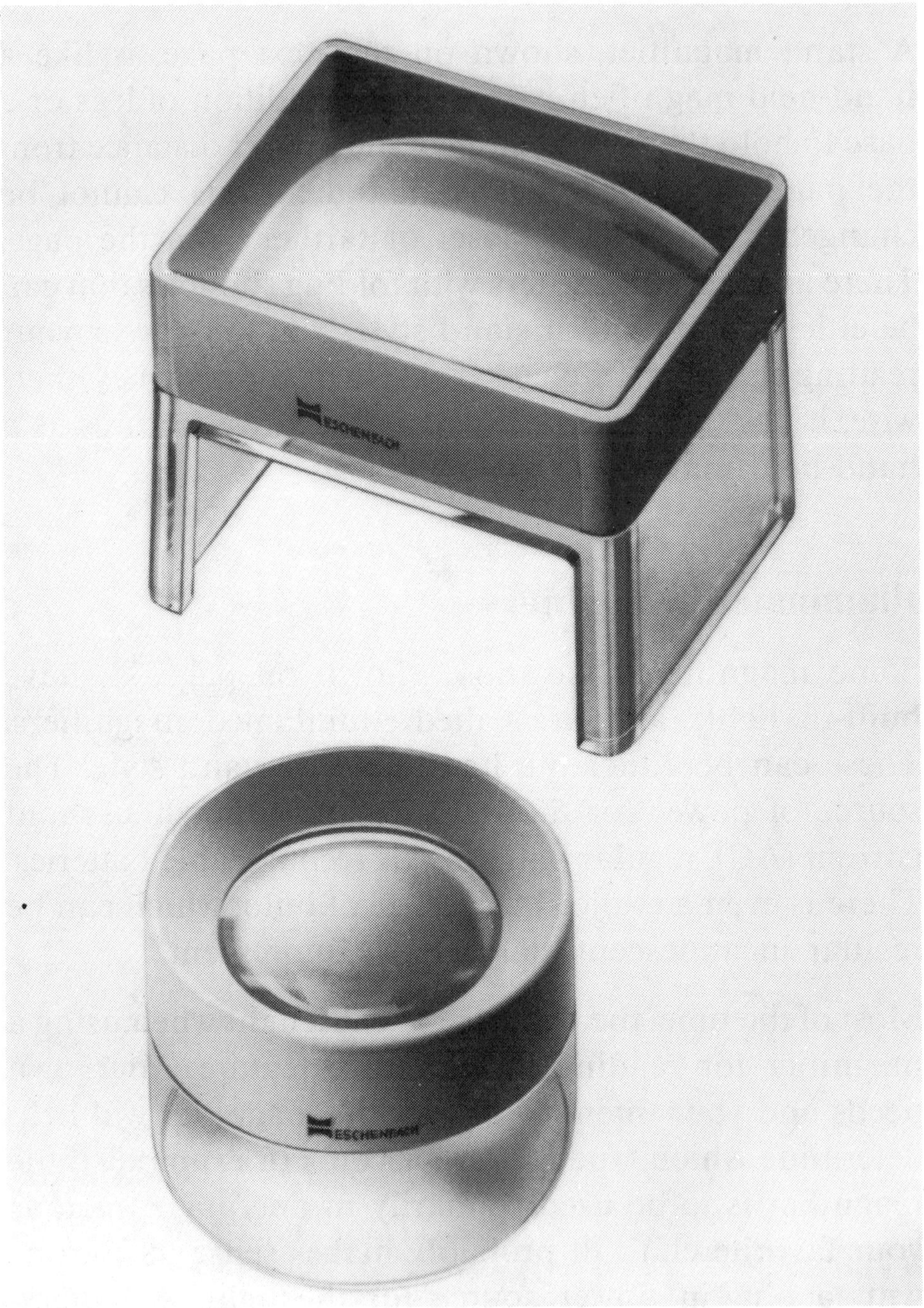

Photo courtesy of Eschenbach Optik of America

Stand magnifiers.

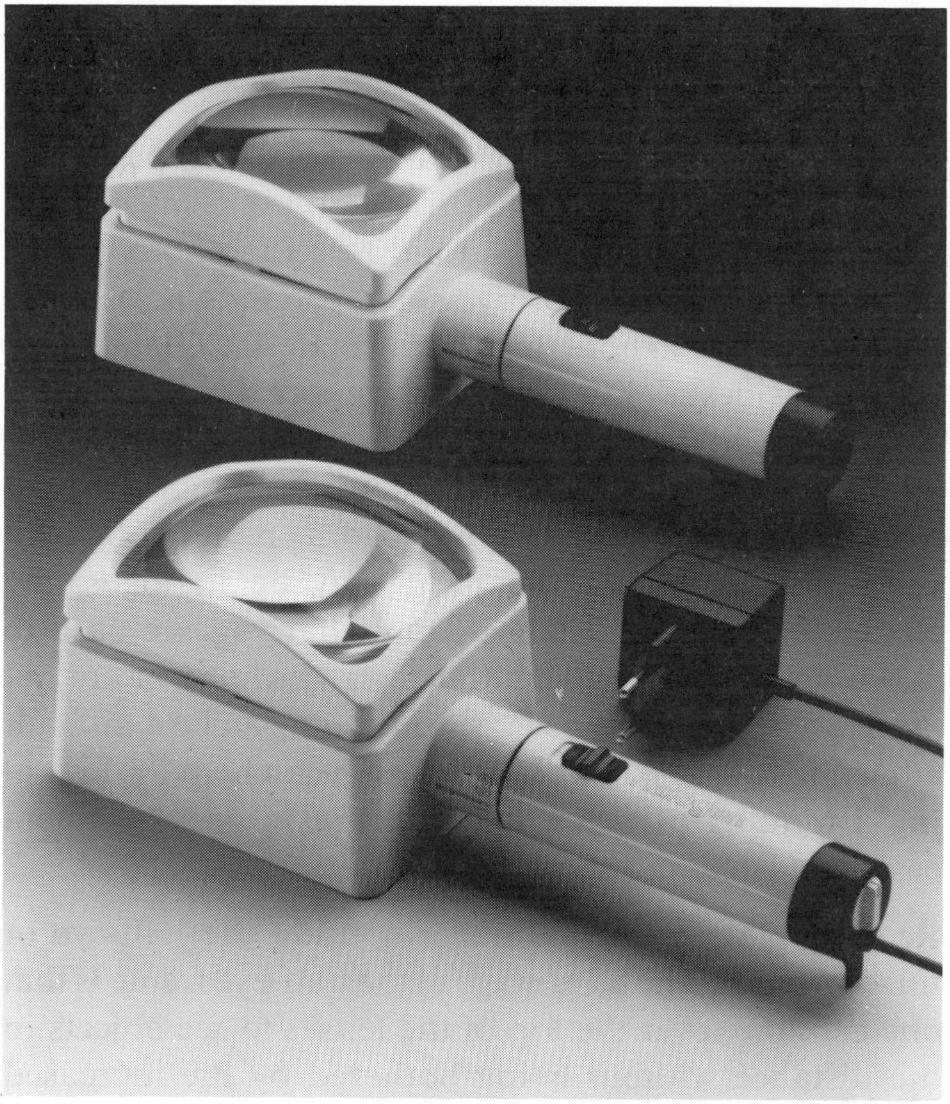

Photo courtesy of Eschenbach Optik of America

Illuminated stand magnifiers.

likes. It is important to be able to try different types of lights at the same magnification to see which works best for you.

Reading Glasses

Reading glasses, sometimes called "microscopes," present a good example of the trade-offs one must make when choosing a low vision aid (see the photo on the facing page). On the positive side, reading glasses leave your hands free to hold the reading material. Glasses also offer the widest field of view (how many words or letters you can see at one time) of any optical aid. On the other hand, most people do not like that these high-powered reading glasses require that the reading material be held very close. Although the print may be in focus, the change of reading distance from what you are used to (13–16 inches or 33–40 centimeters) to what you are not used to (2–6 inches or 5–15 centimeters) can be a difficult adjustment. A specialist in low vision can help by designing a training program that will make the adjustment easier and reading more successful.

Reading glasses can be made in either the half-eye or full-view style. The advantage of the half-eye frame is that one can look over the top of the lenses to see objects in the distance without being bothered by the increased blurriness of looking through the lenses.

Loupes and Visors

There are several different types of loupes and visors available to people with low vision (see the photo on

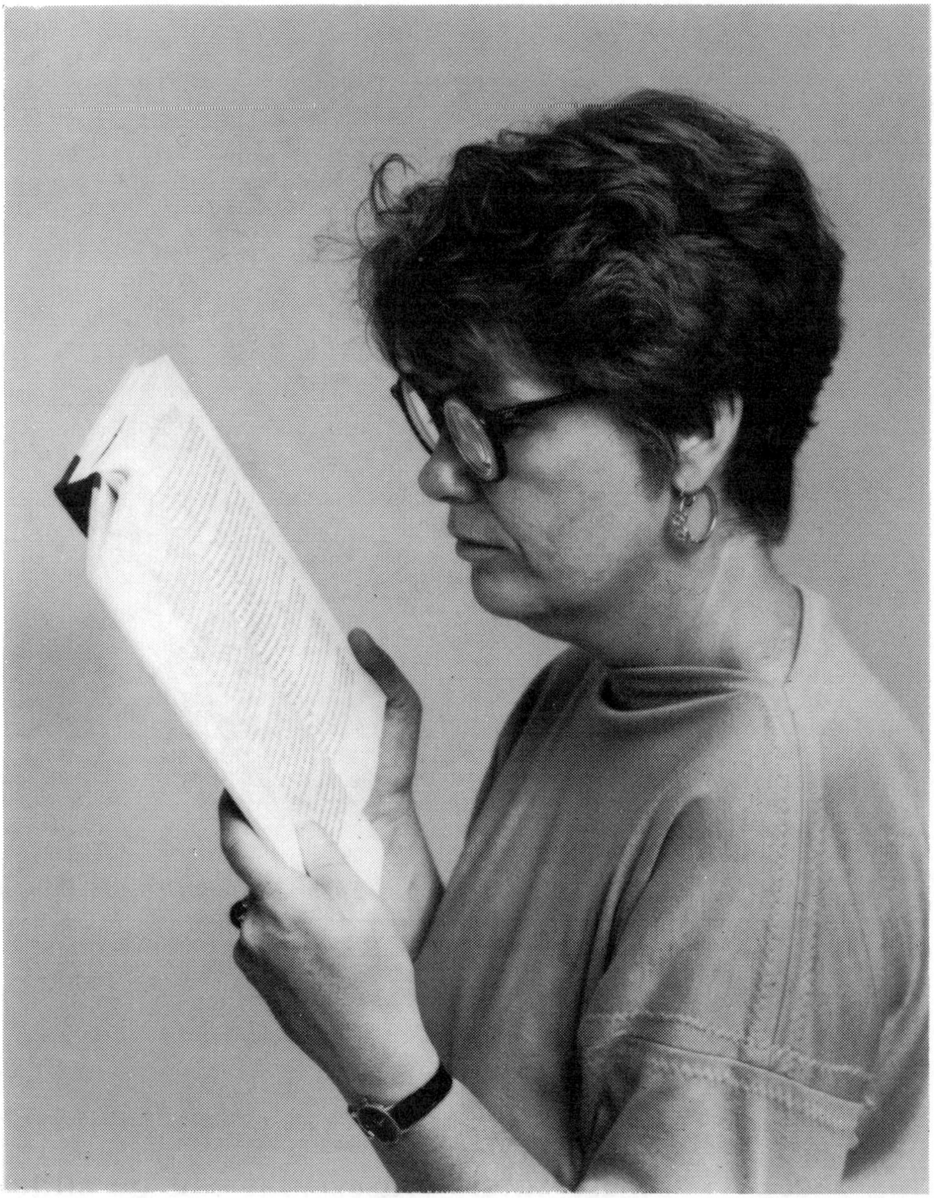

Photo courtesy of Designs For Vision, Inc.

Reading glasses (ClearImage II).

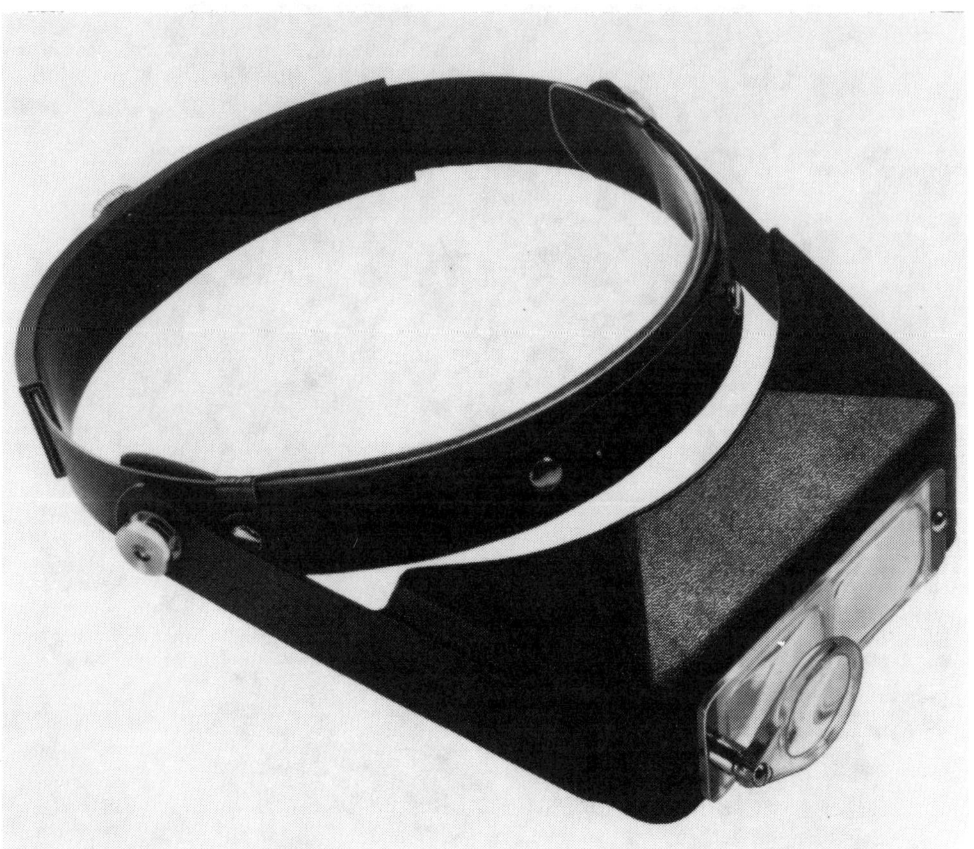

Photo courtesy Donegan Optical

Optivisor, with loupe.

this page). These are single lenses that can be either clipped onto your glasses or are supported by a frame that is attached to a head strap, positioning the lens a few inches in front of the glasses. Although the field of view can be small and the headgear cumbersome, these aids are usually inexpensive and can be flipped out of the way when not in use.

INVOICE NO.: CT-1411

WISCONSIN COUNCIL OF THE BLIND, INC.
354 West Main Street
Madison, Wisconsin 53703
(608) 255-1166

Sold To:

Irv Johnson
1214 Ravine
Janesville, WI 53545

Shipped To:

Same

DATE	DATE SHIPPED	SHIPPED VIA PARCEL POST
3/30/93	03/30/93	
TERMS	FEDERAL I.D. NUMBER	ORDER NUMBER
	39-0977746	

QUANTITY	DESCRIPTION	UNIT PRICE	AMOUNT
1	BL-310 Coping With Lo Vision book	$17.00d	$17.00
			Tax-$.85
			Total- $17.85

ALL SALES ARE FINAL

Reading Telescopes

Reading telescopes, like those on page 78, are low vision aids that are generally considered to be more difficult to use than the previously mentioned devices. This aid consists of one or two small telescopes mounted in a frame and worn like a pair of glasses. For those who are attempting to do a task at about an arm's length, this aid can be extremely useful. Such activities include reading a computer screen, sewing, or woodworking.

There are many different types of reading telescopes. Some are very small and can be mounted in a pair of regular glasses. These can be placed in the bottom portion of the lenses about where the bifocal is usually placed, so you can look over the top of the telescope when you don't need it. This type of telescope, allowing you to look through it or above or below it, is a "bioptic telescope."

Other types of reading telescopes are mounted in the middle of the lenses, so you look through them all the time. This usually makes the aid easier to use. However, it is not possible to walk around safely while wearing this type of reading telescope.

Other variations include a choice between a telescope that can be focused for different distances or having the focus set for one specific distance. Some telescopes allow you to change the distance where an object will be in focus by turning one end of the telescope. Others are focused for distant objects, but can be made to work for reading by placing a special lens, or "reading cap," over the front lens of the telescope. It then becomes a fixed-focus reading telescope.

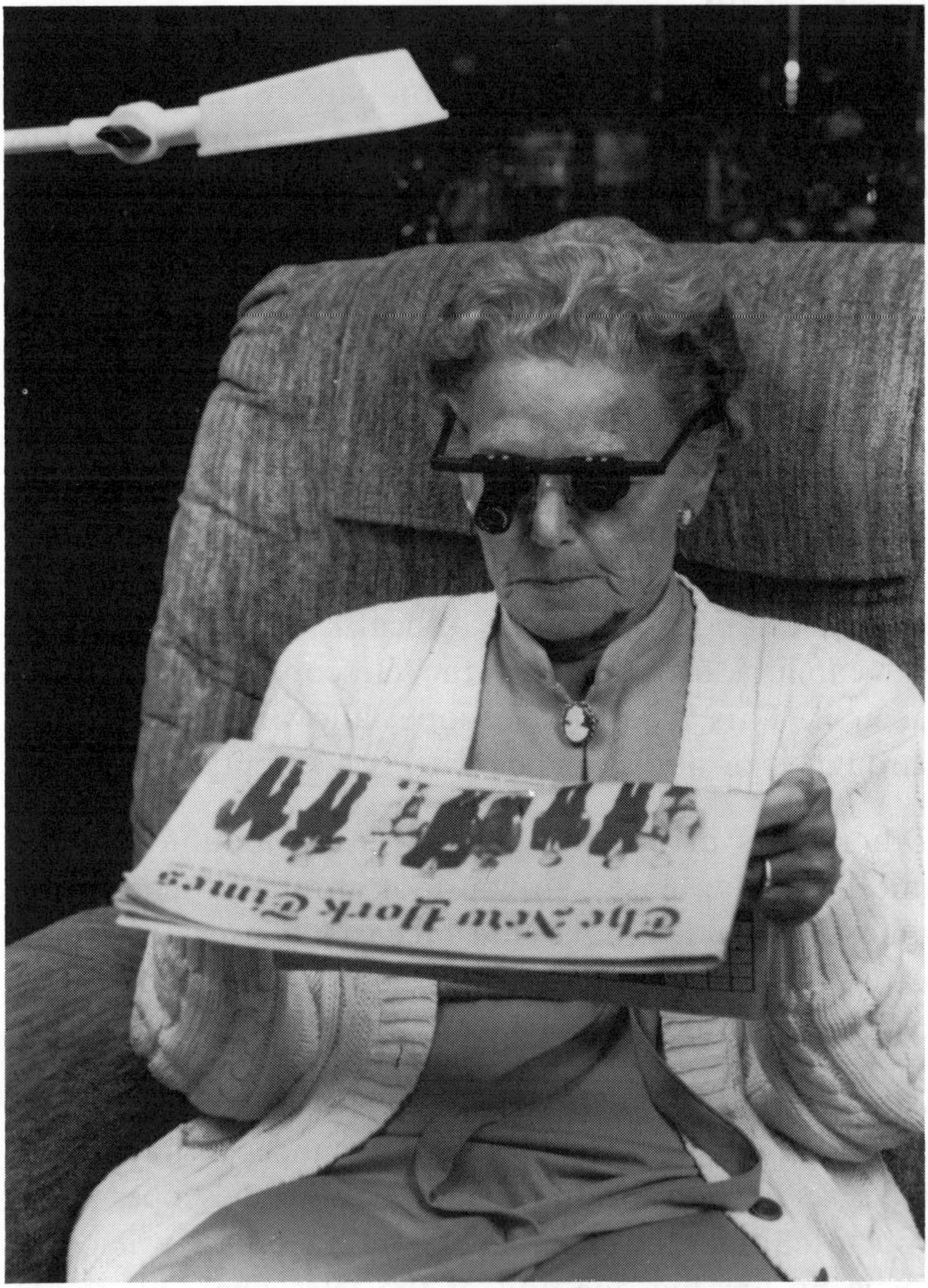

Photo courtesy of Eschenbach Optik of America

Reading telescopes.

The advantages of a reading telescope include allowing the user to have high magnification of an object at an intermediate, or "arm's length," distance, freeing the hands from holding the device. One major disadvantage is that the area you can see at a given time (field of view) can be very limited. Another disadvantage is that the distance between the object being looked at and your telescope must not change (shallow depth of field) or the image will go out of focus. Also, if you shake, cough, or take a deep breath, the thing you are looking at may appear very blurry until you are still again. In other words, you must keep your head still while using the aid. Despite the drawbacks, reading telescopes can be helpful to a person who needs magnification at middle distance.

Telescopes

The only low vision aids that will improve vision for objects in the distance are telescopes (see the photo on the next page). A telescope is a series of lenses lined up at specific distances from each other. A telescope for one eye is called a monocular and a telescope for two eyes is called a binocular. Some telescopes focus only in the distance (Galilean) while others can be focused to a distance as close as 8 inches (Keplerian).

Telescopes can be mounted in a frame to be worn on the head, and, like the reading telescopes, these can be mounted directly in front of the eyes or positioned just out of the direct line of vision (bioptic).

Hand-held telescopes are another type of aid. Most people are familiar with binoculars, field glasses, or opera

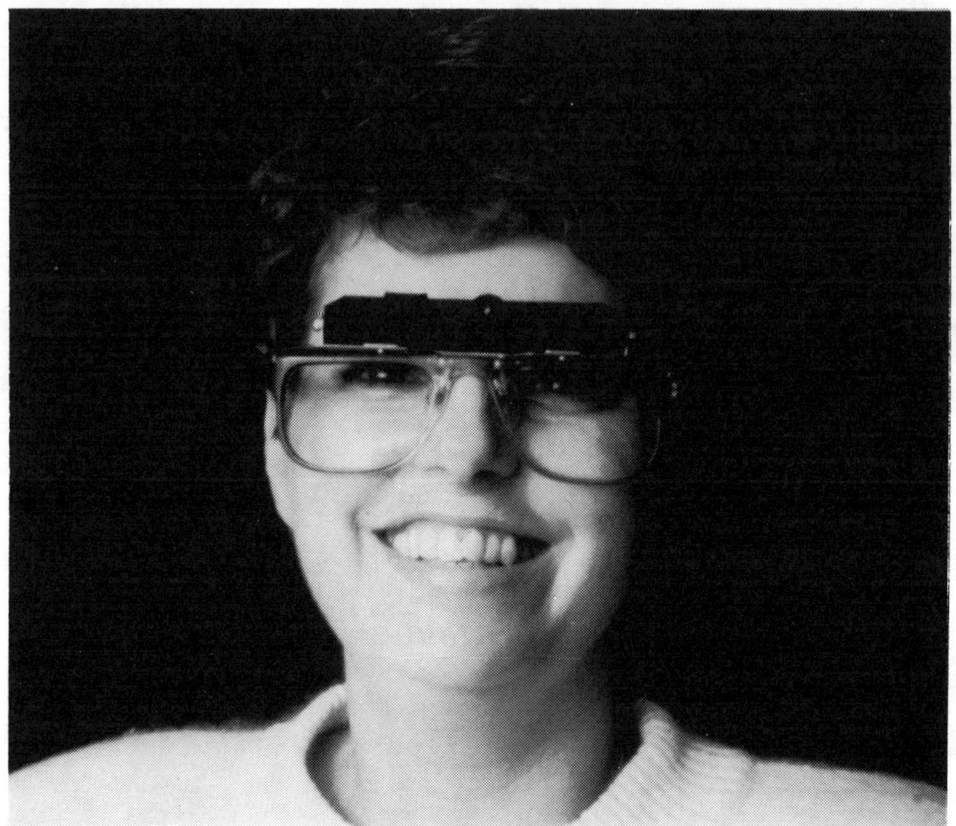

Photo courtesy Ocutech, Inc.

Ocutech VES, spectacle-mounted telescope.

glasses. In fact, many people with low vision discover that these are more useful than ever for watching sporting events, wildlife, or concerts and plays. Although some binoculars are small and lightweight, many people prefer to use a monocular, which is smaller, lighter, and easier to carry. Many monoculars on the market today are about the size of an adult's thumb and can be easily carried in a pocket or purse. They are very useful for reading street signs (when walking), house numbers, or destination signs on public transportation.

Telescopes can be difficult to use because they offer only a small area which can be seen at one time (field of view) and because you must hold the telescope very steady. This is usually difficult to do at first, but you can gain skill with instruction and practice. Because of this limitation, which increases with the power of the telescope, monoculars and binoculars that magnify more than eight times (8×) are not routinely recommended.

Video Magnifiers

A closed-circuit television or a video magnifier like the one on page 82 is a small television camera with a zoom close-up lens that can enlarge a picture of print or a photograph from such material as a book, magazine, newspaper, or letter onto a special television screen (monitor). The user can make the image as big as necessary (up to 60 times on some models) and can also turn black letters on a white background into white letters on a black background (reverse polarity). Many people find that this high contrast image is much easier to see.

This aid allows a person to sit at a table and read print at a normal distance and it offers very high magnification. Some models have special line marker features that can make following a line of print easier. The main disadvantage of this aid is its cost. Basic models from many companies start between $2,000 and $3,000. For some this amount of money is beyond their budget, but others find that the money saved on other activities, such as an automobile and its insurance and upkeep, allows them to afford such a purchase. Many libraries, retirement com-

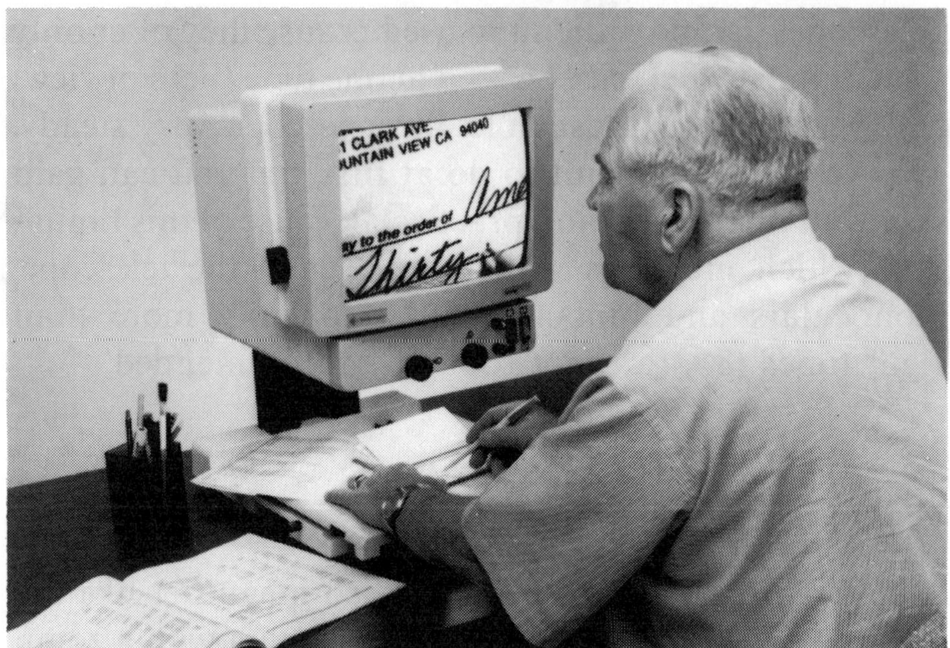

Photo courtesy of TeleSensory, Inc.

Video magnifier.

plexes, and senior centers make video magnifiers available by placing one in a convenient common area.

Aids For Visual Field Loss

Some people do not have the problem of blurry vision, but can benefit from some optical aids. These are people who have lost their side, or peripheral, vision. They may have lost vision in the top, bottom, and side areas of their vision and have "tunnel vision," (as in glaucoma or retinitis pigmentosa) or they may have lost the left or right side of their vision (such as a hemianopia after a stroke). Although they often can see details, their vision is like looking down a narrow tube. Large amounts of magnification are not always helpful for these people because their field of view is so small. There are two basic types of aids to help people who have lost a large amount of their side vision. These are prisms and reverse telescopes.

Prisms

Prisms are used to expand visual field *awareness* in people who have lost side vision. This should not be confused with the use of prisms in low vision reading glasses allowing one to use both eyes together when holding the material closely. Nor should it be misunderstood as the use of prism lenses to bend light entering the eye onto the healthier part of the retina. The prisms used for expanding visual field awareness are thin pieces of plastic called **Fresnel** (freh NEL) prisms. They are applied to the inside of the lens of the user's regular glasses just outside of the working visual field, usually on the side nearest the temple, or bow, of the glasses (see the photo on page 84). When the user is looking straight ahead, the prism cannot be seen. However, glancing to the side the prism is positioned on and looking through it makes objects on the side appear to be more directly in front of the viewer. This can eliminate the need to constantly turn the head to check on what is to one's side.

As with other low vision aids, the use of prisms in this way has positive and negative features. Although it can add up to 15 degrees of visual field awareness, the Fresnel prism can be confusing and disorienting as one glances in and out of regular vision and the prism. To use this aid effectively requires training from an experienced professional.

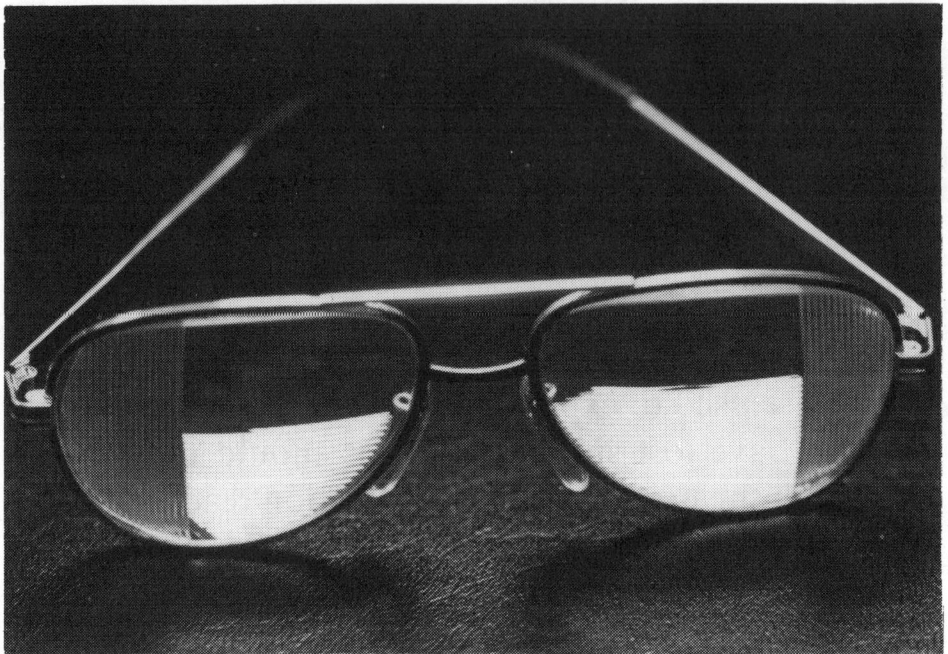

Photo courtesy Dr. Stephen Kessler

Fresnel prisms on lower and outside portion of lenses.

Reverse Telescopes

As a child, did you ever play with binoculars and look through them backwards? You may remember that everything looked small and far away. What you may not have noticed is that you could see a larger area. This is an example of how **reverse telescopes** work (see the photo on the facing page). Earlier in this chapter you learned about telescopes that could be mounted in either the center of the eyeglass lens or in the bioptic position, allowing the user to see with his or her regular vision. You then obtain the benefits of the telescope by glancing up or down into the telescopic lens.

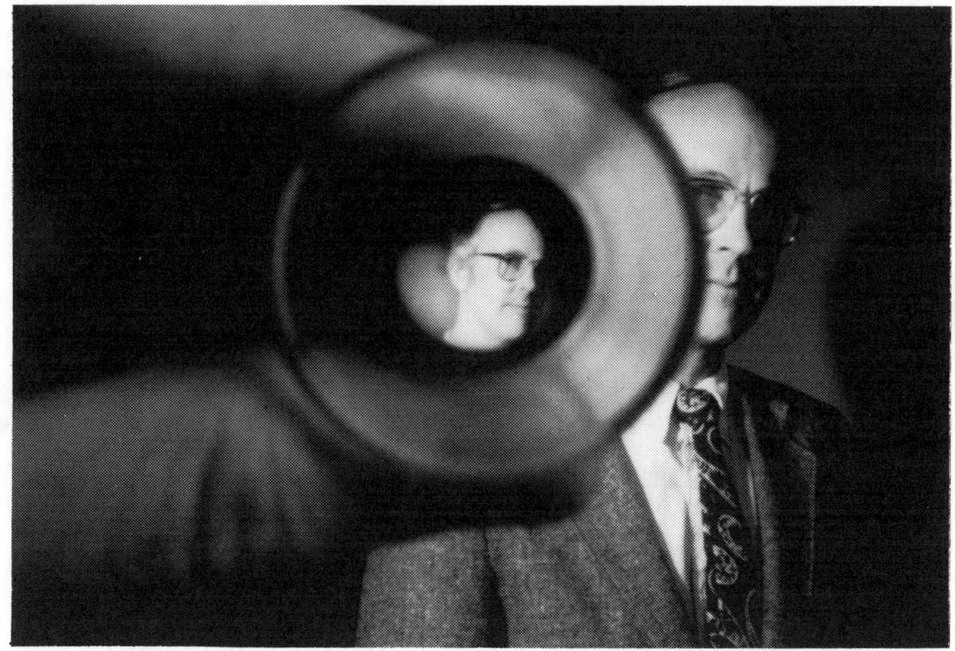

Photo courtesy Ocutech, Inc.

Visual field minifier (reverse telescope).

The same arrangement works with the telescope reversed, or turned backwards. The field of view is increased and this saves the user from moving the head from side to side to see what is outside of the small visual field. However, because everything seen through the reverse telescope is smaller than it really is, you must have good visual acuity to benefit from this aid.

Nonoptical Aids

There are many helpful aids or devices for people with low vision that do not use lenses. These are nonoptical aids. Nonoptical aids can include large-print books, talking clocks and watches, and specially marked pill boxes. Lights and reading stands are nonoptical aids that are important for people who are trying to read with low vision aids.

Lights

To see better, most people with low vision need more light than typical readers or viewers. This is particularly true for those with age-related maculopathy. Those who don't need more light often need to be able to control the amount and direction of the light they are using. Although individual needs will vary, there are basic rules for using light when you have low vision.

How Much Light?

Typically, when you think of increasing the amount of light in your home, you think of replacing your light bulbs with higher wattage bulbs. As long as one does not exceed the wattage limits of the light fixture, this will probably help to brighten rooms. But, when it comes to reading with low vision, it is more important to **get the light closer to the page**. In other words, increasing the size of the bulb in your shaded lamp on the end table or in the ceiling fixture will not help you with reading nearly as much as using a regular wattage bulb in a lamp that you can place close to the page.

What Kind of Lamp?

Your lamp should have a gooseneck or flexible arm for positioning close to the material you are reading. It is hard to read if the light is in front of you and shining in your face. The lamp should also have a shield that deflects the light down onto the page. This will prevent you from having to squint to avoid discomfort from the extra, bright light.

Bulbs

Your choice of what type of bulb to use is up to you. Different people prefer different types of illumination. Your choices include:

1. *Incandescent* — easy to find, inexpensive; but can get very hot.
2. *Fluorescent* — very little heat; double-tube fluorescent can eliminate shadows.
3. *Halogen* — higher cost but lower electricity use than incandescent; very bright light, high-heat output.
4. *Full spectrum* — a "grow–light" that provides a balanced light similar to sunlight.
5. *Compact fluorescent* — higher initial cost, but energy-efficient, low heat.

When using a bulb that gets very hot, be cautious when touching the parts of the lamp around the bulb because they may also be very hot. Also, do not use a bulb of higher wattage than the fixture manufacturer specifies.

Clipboards and Reading Stands

Although they are not the most sophisticated or glamorous low vision aids, clipboards and reading stands are among the most useful. Because of the unique requirements of reading with low vision, it is usually easier to read with either of these.

Clipboards

A clipboard is especially useful for giving you a firm, flat surface on which to move your stand magnifier or for giving a supportive backing to flimsy papers. If you are able to read the newspaper with your low vision aid, it is doubtful that you will be able to hold it wide open as you might have done when fully sighted. By folding the paper to the size of a clipboard, you will be able to work more efficiently and easily. A clipboard is also useful for single sheets of paper, such as letters and bills.

Reading Stands

A reading stand, like the one on the facing page, is particularly useful for people who use high-powered low vision aids with a very short working distance and/or a very shallow depth of field. Such aids require the reading material to be held steady. Also, a stand can relieve neck and back strain from leaning over a page or book lying flat on a table.

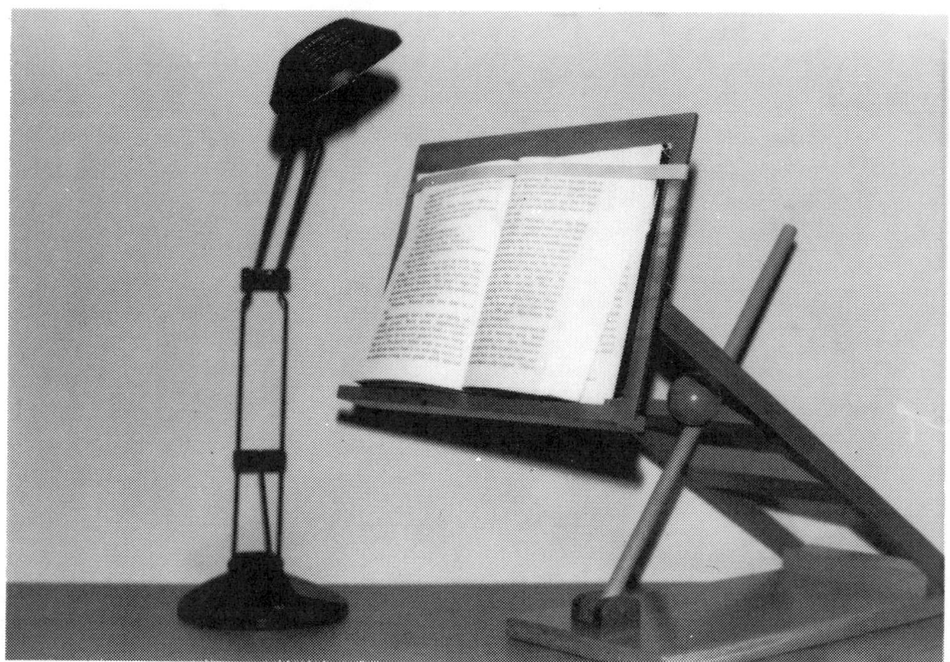

Photo courtesy Marshall Flax.

Reading stand and flex-arm light.

Although there are many types of optical and nonoptical aids available to people with low vision, each has its own set of characteristics for its own specific job. This is the same for kitchen appliances or tools in the workshop. Knowledge of the different types of aids and each one's purpose will help you choose the one(s) best for you.

Chapter 13

Eccentric Viewing

Eccentric viewing is the name of a technique for people who have lost their central vision. They can use the procedure to help themselves get the greatest possible use out of their remaining vision. While the word "eccentric" has come to be used to describe someone who is odd or peculiar, the first dictionary meaning is "off-center." The technique of eccentric viewing is learning how to use your off-center vision.

Central Blind Spot

People who have damage to their eyes from age-related maculopathy will usually have a central blind spot (scotoma) (skoe TOME ah) in their vision. This means that wherever they look, the portion of the picture that is in the middle will be missing, blurry, and/or distorted. When you look at print on a page, the middle of a word might be missing. When you look at someone's face, it is hard to see their features. It is a little bit like going to a movie theater to find that a large part of the center of the screen is missing. Whatever part of the movie scene falls on the missing area of the screen can't be seen by the audience.

Some people perceive this blind spot as a distinct spot or shape in their vision. Others only see a blur wherever they look.

Enhancement Techniques

To get the most out of your remaining vision when a central blind spot is present requires learning to use your side vision (peripheral vision) in a different way.

One technique that many people find helpful is to think of the area that you can see as though it were the face of a large clock. Like all clocks, 12 is at the top, 6 is at the bottom, 3 is on the right and 9 is on the left. In the middle you can imagine a spot where the big hand and the little hand are joined together.

To use your eccentric vision, you need to discover the location of your area(s) of best remaining vision. Do this by using the clock technique.

1. Begin by sitting in a comfortable chair about 10 feet away from a familiar object (the "target"). A door knob, a small picture on the wall, or a kitchen wall clock are possibilities.

2. Cover your blurrier eye.

3. Look at your target so it is in the middle of the "clock." If you are doing this properly, the target should seem to disappear or get blurrier. This is because you are lining it up with your central blind spot, or scotoma.

4. Now look slightly above the target, or at "12:00." Does the target become a little easier to see? If so, practice this a few times. By making a slight change in where you are looking you may be able to make the target appear and disappear. If looking slightly above the target didn't make a big change in what you could see, you need to try a different area. Even if the 12:00 position worked, you should complete this exercise to learn if you have other "islands of good remaining vision" or areas that work even better.

5. Next, relocate the target in the center of your vision so it is blurry. Now try the 3:00 position as you did with the 12:00 position in number 4, above.
6. Continue this process at the 6:00 and 9:00 positions. If these prove to be helpful, you can chose the one or ones that seem to be easiest to use and practice with targets of different sizes and at different distances. For example, you might find that when you wish to see someone's face more clearly, you can do so by looking at an ear or above the forehead.
7. If the four basic positions do not prove to be helpful, try going around the imaginary clock of your vision again. This time, try the hours between those that you just tried. For example, try 1:30, 4:30, 7:30, and 10:30.

Remember, to see the target best, you must not look directly at it. This can be hard to remember and will take some practice.

Practice the technique of eccentric viewing regularly and you will soon become so used to it that you will forget that you are doing it.

This technique will not restore your vision, but it can help you to get the most use out of your remaining vision. It will not damage your eyes in any way to do these exercises, nor will it make any change for the better in the eyes themselves. If you are not able to get eccentric viewing to work for you, consult with your low vision therapist.

Chapter 14

Rehabilitation Teaching

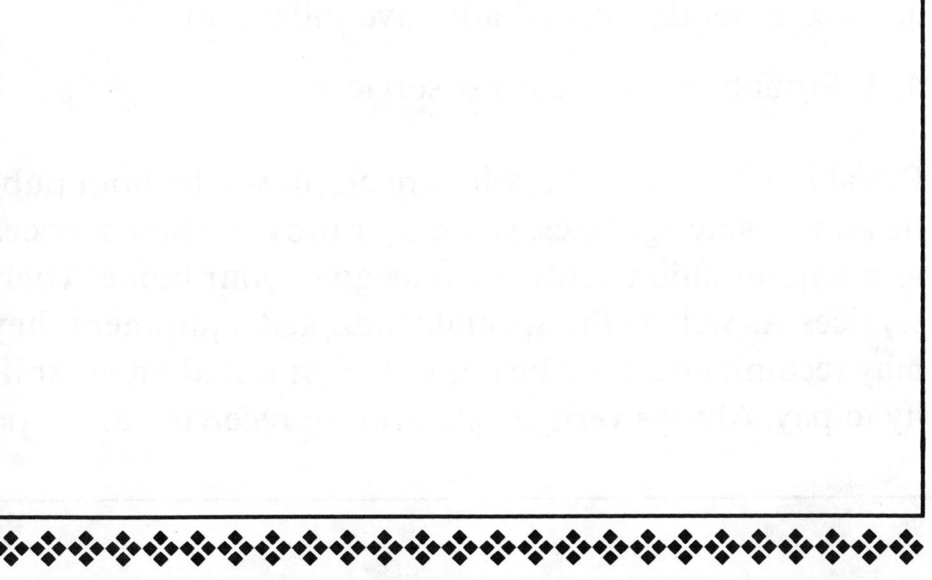

As you have read, most people first learn of the magnitude of their vision loss from their eye doctor. Naturally the questions patients commonly ask are related to medical concerns and possible cures, not about the availability of rehabilitation services for people who must live with low vision. If your doctor tells you "nothing more can be done," it means that no medical procedure or drug may be expected to improve your vision. If you are told you have a condition that may continue in some way to limit your independent daily activities, you should ask about the availability of rehabilitation teaching services in your area. This chapter reinforces that "something can be done."

The Rehabilitation Teacher

A rehabilitation teacher is a professional who provides:

1. Counseling to help a person and family members adjust to living with low vision;
2. Instruction in a variety of personal skill areas;
3. Recommendations of adaptive aids; and
4. Information and referral services.

Rehabilitation teachers, who are employed by both public and private agencies, will either provide their services in a rehabilitation center or may go to your home. Their services, as well as the specially adapted equipment they may recommend, may be either free or based on an ability to pay. Always verify costs prior to receiving any type of service or adaptive equipment. (See Appendix B for a listing of your state or provincial services for the blind.) In larger metropolitan areas, you may be able to contact more than one service provider to compare their services, approaches, and philosophies before you decide to proceed with the one that most closely meets your needs.

Teaching Process

The rehabilitation teacher will begin a process designed to assist you to adjust to low vision. You may be called a "client" or a "student." Although the steps you will follow may differ based on the agency's policy, the following are the most common steps in the rehabilitation teaching process.

- Eligibility determination
- Assessment of abilities and needs
- Development of an individualized plan of service
- Individual and family counseling
- Recommendations of adaptive aids
- Direct instruction
- Information and referral
- Invitations to support groups

Eligibility

The rehabilitation teacher (or other agency staff member) will determine your eligibility based on their policies. Some agencies merely require that an individual have a vision loss that limits independent functioning, while others will only provide services to legally blind individuals. Typically, you will be asked to complete an application, as well as sign a release form that your eye doctor will complete verifying the cause and extent of your condition. Also, an extensive interview may occur at this stage.

Assessment

The rehabilitation teacher will conduct an assessment of your background, living situation, local support from friends and family, hobbies and interests, and how you are able to handle your everyday needs. This assessment may include both a verbal interview and a demonstration of your daily tasks for evaluation. You may be asked to set your oven dial, address an envelope, read a watch, or measure a cup of flour. You will be asked what leisure activities are important to you. Together, you and the rehabilitation teacher will agree on the specific skill areas needing improvement.

Individualized Plan of Service

After you have been determined eligible for services, and have shown a need to be able to better deal with life's demands, your individual plan of service will be developed. In some instances, you may be required to sign a detailed, written plan of service, whereas in others, the plan may merely be part of a case record. In either circumstance, you should expect to have input on what services you receive. You should also be able to obtain a copy of the plan if you wish.

Counseling

A rehabilitation teacher may provide counseling, both individually and in a group setting, to help you come to terms with your decreased vision. This is not to say that you will be expected to like, or even be totally comfortable, seeing less clearly than before. However, counseling should help you to accept a vision loss for what it is — a situation that you may have to live with and adapt to. You may then be better prepared to live your life more fully despite the vision loss. Counseling will normally be an ongoing aspect of rehabilitation services and may occur at any time you or the rehabilitation teacher feel a need to talk about your concerns.

You can expect that the issues you discuss during counseling, or at any other time with the rehabilitation teacher, will remain confidential.

Family Counseling

As vision loss affects all members of a family, it is important that relatives be encouraged to attend the counseling sessions the rehabilitation teacher provides. The rehabilitation teacher can help your family members better understand what vision loss is, what it's not, and how to best live with it. An important point to remember is that

that most people with low vision want and are usually able to be independent. Family members can learn during counseling sessions how to understand vision loss, how to accept it for what it is, and how to best enable the person with low vision to be independent.

Adapted Aid Recommendations

Depending on your needs and abilities, the rehabilitation teacher may recommend different kinds of specially adapted equipment. Although mail order businesses (see Appendix A for a listing of consumer products catalogs) all sell a wide variety of kitchen timers, for instance, the rehabilitation teacher can help determine the very best one for you. After trying large print, raised print, or talking timers you will be better able to decide which meets your needs. The final decision will be based on your vision, your senses of touch and hearing, your motivation, and your budget. Often, the rehabilitation teacher will be able to provide a "loaner" on a trial basis.

Direct Instruction

A rehabilitation teacher is, of course, a person who teaches. Having low vision causes certain difficulties in many areas of our lives. The following categories list a few examples of the skills needed to accomplish activities of daily living.

Communication Skills

Many people find that their most immediate and ongoing concern after developing a visual loss is a need to continue written communications. Although braille may be the first thing that comes to mind when low vision and communication skills are mentioned, it is not the answer for everyone.

Braille is a raised-dot, touch system of reading and writing used by people who are blind. This system, developed by Louis Braille, a Frenchman who was blind, allows the freedom to learn and communicate. The alphabet, numbers, and punctuation are all represented by varying which of six dots of a braille cell are raised. Braille also employs a form of shorthand by using certain dot combinations (contractions) to stand for whole words.

Although learning braille for extensive reading does take persistence and effort, it is invaluable for those who master it. Even if you are able to make use of low vision therapy, optical aids, and large print, you may find braille to be especially useful for marking, labeling, and taking notes. If you have an interest in learning braille, especially for labeling or playing cards, please ask your rehabilitation teacher for more information.

The rehabilitation teacher can assist you with other communication skills:

- Relearn effective **script writing** using bold marking pens, script-writing templates, and dark-lined paper;
- Learn **record-keeping** or note-taking techniques with less vision;

- Learn **braille** for reading, writing, playing cards, and labeling;
- Become familiar with the use of **large print or talking books** or other library services;
- Use **large print or "talking" equipment** such as computers, tape recorders, and clocks.

Orientation and Mobility Instruction

The rehabilitation teacher can also offer orientation and mobility instruction to help you learn to maintain or regain safe mobility skills. This instruction may include learning how to walk with a sighted guide, learning self-protective techniques, and learning how to locate dropped objects. Rehabilitation teachers may teach you ways to get in and out of cars effectively and use stairs safely. You may also learn to develop your other senses, such as hearing and touch. When necessary, the rehabilitation teacher may refer you to an orientation and mobility instructor to learn safe and efficient outdoor travel skills, such as crossing streets with the use of a white cane. (See Chapter 15 for more on orientation and mobility.) A discussion on the merits of a referral to a dog guide school should also be part of a comprehensive orientation and mobility program.

Personal Management

Personal management includes learning new ways to handle all your personal needs with less vision. The following skills are included in a program of personal management:

- Learning how to continue **grooming** tasks, such as shaving, nail care, or applying makeup;
- **Money management** including learning ways to identify coins and paper money;
- Proper **table etiquette**;
- **Organization skills** necessary in everyday life to simplify the location and identification of personal items such as clothing, medications, and tools.

Home Management

A program of home-management skills includes instruction to assist you in better dealing with the demands of managing a household. A person with low vision will learn different and better ways to:

- **Organize** his or her belongings;
- **Identify** household items by special large print, bold, bright, or raised markings;
- Handle routine **cleaning**;
- Make minor **repairs**;
- **Launder and mend** clothing;
- Safely and efficiently **prepare meals**.

Some of the specially adapted home-management items you will see are large- or raised-print timers, large-print labels for canned goods, materials for marking and labeling, large-print or recorded cookbooks, slicing and measuring guides, and sewing needle threaders, to name a few.

Leisure Time and Recreational Activities

The rehabilitation teacher you work with will offer assistance with techniques for the following recreational activities:

- Continuing with **crafts or handwork;**
- Using large-print, raised-print, or braille **table games**;
- Using large-print or braille **playing cards**;
- Enjoying the crowd atmosphere of **spectator sports**, possibly with a friend or group providing vivid descriptions of the action as needed;
- Descriptive video, a means of describing the video portion of television broadcasts. For example, the describer explains subtle facial gestures, describes the setting, and gives the overall visual picture of what the fully sighted viewer sees, but the person with low vision misses.

There are organizations devoted to encouraging people with low vision to continue being active in recreational activities. These include Blind Outdoor Leisure Development (BOLD), the American Blind Bowling Association, and Ski for Light. See Appendix A for more on recreational opportunities.

Group tours, often sponsored by rehabilitation centers, senior groups, or travel agencies, offer a great opportunity to be socially involved while experiencing new places or activities. Transportation, meals, and lodging may be provided as part of a convenient package.

Information and Referral

During the course of receiving rehabilitation teaching services, other needs and concerns, not directly a part of the rehabilitation plan of service, may develop. At such a point, it is the responsibility of the rehabilitation teacher to give information on important community resources and to make the referral when needed.

Peer Support Groups

Many people with low vision benefit from involvement in peer or self-help support groups coordinated by a rehabilitation teacher, an agency, or, sometimes, a person affected by loss of vision. Attending support groups may help you overcome a common perception among people with a recent vision loss — that they are the only one with the condition and nobody understands what they are going through. If no such group is available in your area, contact the Lighthouse National Center For Vision and Aging (see Appendix A) for its published resource directory on support groups for people with low vision, your state's services for the blind, or a rehabilitation teacher for information on starting one.

Although your eye doctor may not be able to restore your vision, there is something that can be done. Obtaining the services of a qualified rehabilitation teacher is one of the best things you can do for yourself.

Chapter 15

Orientation and Mobility

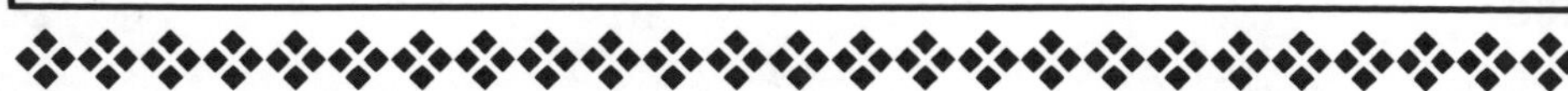

The Problem of Getting Around

For many people who lose vision, the loss of the ability to travel independently and safely is a severe blow. A simple trip to the grocery store that previously was a routine outing that hardly required much thought may now seem to be an epic journey filled with fear and embarrassment. Some of the reasons for this anxiety may include:

- Crossing busy streets;
- Navigating around obstacles;
- Detecting curbs, stairs, and other level changes;
- Accidently bumping into people.

These concerns may cause people to go out only when necessary. This, in turn, is likely to increase their feelings of isolation.

Driving a car, an essential form of transportation for many Americans, is often out of the question. For those who live in rural areas or small towns, this can mean increased isolation from friends, neighbors, and basic services. Using public transportation, when available, may seem impossible to a person who cannot see the number of a bus or train.

Orientation and Mobility

Orientation and mobility, or O and M, is the instructional area teaching people who are blind or visually impaired how to travel safely, efficiently, and as independently as possible. Techniques include using the arm of a fully sighted person or using a white cane (typhlocane). Basic instruction can be provided by either an O and M specialist or a rehabilitation teacher. Advanced instruction should be taught by a certified orientation and mobility instructor.

There are many levels of O and M instruction that can be provided at many different points in one's rehabilitation process. One of the most common is instructing people how to move safely in their homes. This may include learning to go up and down stairs, locate objects, and find doorways.

Another area is covered by teaching the sighted guide technique for traveling in unfamiliar areas. This is having **the person who is visually impaired hold the arm of a sighted person** — not, as often thought, the other way around. For the person with a visual impairment, this is one of the most important points to remember for safe travel. Although it is common for the sighted person to want to take the arm of the person with a vision impairment and push or pull them through the environment, it should be the visually impaired person who holds on and follows slightly behind. With proper instruction and practice, a person who is visually impaired can safely use the sighted guide to go in and out of doorways, up and down stairs, and through crowds in unfamiliar areas.

The White Cane

Instruction in the use of a cane for independent travel may not be needed by those who have a significant amount of remaining vision. Many people are unwilling to take up the use of a tool that broadcasts to those around them that they have a visual impairment. Others choose to not use a cane, as they see the use as a symbol that their vision is permanently impaired. Still others fear that a white cane will label them as an easy target for criminals. But even with all the sincere reasons people decide not to use a cane for traveling, there are still many times when a cane can be very useful.

Although there are people who wish to keep their impairment from being known, many others find security in carrying a cane to let others know that they may not see very well. This is especially helpful when crossing streets.

There are laws in all 50 states requiring that a motorist yield to a person who is crossing a street using a white cane (or a dog guide). A white cane can alert others that the person using the cane may need extra time and may not readily see some vehicles. However, the person crossing a street using a cane needs to remain alert. It is unwise to solely rely on motorists to see the cane and respond appropriately.

A person who has received professional instruction in the use of a cane for independent travel should be able to detect curbs, steps and other drop-offs, and walk in unfamiliar areas with greater confidence. This enables the individual to pay more attention to the surrounding environment instead of focusing on the ground at one's feet.

Other Help

An orientation and mobility instructor can help you with necessary new strategies for traveling. For example, based on the position of the sun, the temperature and the general weather, what is the best time of day for you to travel and what are the best routes? Do hats and sunglasses help or hinder your ability to get around? Are there ways to position your body to get the most out of your remaining vision?

Instruction in orientation and mobility can help you use the "rules" about the outdoor environment, such as the system by which buildings are numbered and how many steps between the sidewalk and the curb in business or residential neighborhoods. The training can also help you cope with the lack of "rules" for indoor environments, such as unexpected steps up or down, escalators, or revolving doors.

It is not possible to teach these skills in this book. If you are interested in receiving instruction to increase your safety and independence, contact your nearest rehabilitation center or state agency for the blind (Appendix B).

Driving With Low Vision

As previously mentioned, the loss of the ability to drive a vehicle is one of the most difficult adjustments for many people with low vision. This loss of independent mobility can contribute to increased feelings of social isolation and may cause conflicts in families. Conflicts may occur when a person who didn't do much of the driving must now take over that job. However, there **may** be an option for people with low vision who wish to continue to drive.

Each state or province has its own rules for the amount of vision (how clear it is [acuity] and how much can be seen [visual field]) that is necessary to obtain a driver's license. If you are interested in learning if you can continue to drive, contact your department of motor vehicles and obtain a copy of the code pertaining to the visual requirements for driving. Next, you should talk about your own situation to a professional in the field of low vision to learn how your abilities correspond with the code requirements. You should receive careful and patient answers to your questions so that you will know exactly where you stand.

In some states, people with low vision are allowed to drive with small telescopes mounted in the lenses of their glasses. While the driver relies primarily on his or her "blurry" vision for most driving tasks, the telescope is available for quickly spotting objects that cannot be positively identified. You should check with your department of motor vehicles *and* your low vision professional to learn more about the regulations that apply to you and your area.

Chapter 16

Community Resources to Cope with Vision Loss

Although coping with low vision is a highly individual experience, it is not something that should be done alone or without professional help. What follows are some of the main resources people with low vision may rely on to obtain rehabilitation and community support. These resources can be beneficial in helping people cope with their loss and develop the skills and abilities required to continue a participatory role in their community. By contacting your state's services for the blind (Appendix B), you may obtain current information on the following resources. As eligibility criteria, costs, and other policies will vary by agency, it's best to ask questions before you agree to receive assistance.

Rehabilitation Services

Federal, state, and provincial governments provide a variety of rehabilitation services for people who are mentally or physically disabled, including, of course, those who have visual impairments or are legally blind. Most of these services are jointly funded (80 percent federal/20 percent state) and are managed by each state's vocational rehabilitation agency or, for people with visual impairments, separate state or provincial services for the blind. (See Appendix B for a list of state and provincial services for the blind.)

Employment

Joint funding from the U.S. Department of Education, Rehabilitation Services Administration (RSA), and each state helps provide counseling, financial assistance for the purchase of tools and payment of tuition or training fees, and job placement services to individuals who are disabled. The goal of these services is to help individuals acquire job skills that will lead to employment.

Independent Living

In addition to employment-related assistance, a variety of independent living services are also available for people with low vision. These supportive services help individuals maintain or enhance their current independent lifestyle. Based on your income and the source of the service, there may be a charge.

Rehabilitation Teaching Services

Rehabilitation teaching services assist people who are blind or have visual impairments to maintain or increase their independence. These specialized services may be available through your state's services for the blind and may also be provided by private agencies. (See Appendix B for a list of state services and Chapter 14 for more information on rehabilitation teaching.)

Rehabilitation Centers

State-Funded Centers

Rehabilitation centers for people who are blind or visually impaired are similar to schools, by offering an intensive schedule of classes outside of an individual's home. The range of classes offered includes a variety of rehabilitation skills as well as the use of high-technology, such as talking computers. In addition to the location of the instruction, the center-based services differ from home-based by providing more intense instruction, a daily class schedule, and a wide range of classes available. Although most centers have lodging on the premises, local students may commute daily. There may be a charge for attending this type of intensive educational program. Contact your state's services for the blind to inquire if a rehabilitation center is near you. (See Appendix B.)

Private Rehabilitation Centers

Private rehabilitation agencies for the blind are found in many large metropolitan areas. These include the Lighthouse programs and those funded by Lion's Clubs and other service organizations. The services offered may include the same range of adjustment programs as offered by state agencies and will often be available both at a center and in an individual's home. There may be a fee for these services. You can check for the availability of private agencies in your community by calling your state's services for the blind (see Appendix B) or by checking the listing under "Blind" or "Rehabilitation" in the Yellow Pages phone book.

Services for Older Persons

In every community in the United States, services available through funding from the Federal Older Americans

Act may cover many of the support needs of older people who are visually impaired. These services are available to people age 60 and older on an ability to pay basis. The services you might receive can include one, several, or all of the following, based on your needs:

- Information and referral services;
- Nutritious meals at senior centers, community centers, or other locations;
- Home-delivered meals (if your health limits your participation at a group meal site);
- Benefits counseling (to help get through the red tape of government and private services such as health care, insurance, and Social Security, to name a few);
- Transportation;
- Health assistance in your home;
- Homemaker services or chore services.

Contact your local aging office for further information. (See "Aging Services" or "Area Agency on Aging" under the government listing in your phone book.)

State Aging Services

Your state aging office or the Area Agency on Aging office may provide additional services to assist an individual to remain in one's own home despite certain health limitations. There is a broad range of supportive programs and services administered by the "aging network," which includes benefit counseling specialists, nutrition programs (both at group meal sites and "Meals-On-Wheels" for homebound individuals), information and referral, transportation programs, and senior center and/or drop-in centers. These programs and services are for individuals 60 and older and are based on an ability to pay. Increasingly, aging program staff are becoming aware of the visually impaired and blind older population and are making efforts to extend their services to people with low vision.

Senior Citizen Centers

Senior citizen centers provide a unique opportunity for communal meals as well as socialization to enhance one's lifestyle. Many senior centers offer educational, recreational, and social opportunities for older people including ceramics classes, billiards tournaments, bingo, exercise classes, and preventive health screenings, to name a few.

Support Groups

Increasing numbers of support groups for people with low vision are forming at local senior centers. These support groups often meet monthly or semimonthly, with a social as well as an educational focus. Membership in the group may be free of charge, through a voluntary contribution, or with a fixed dues structure. (See the Lighthouse National Center For Vision and Aging in Appendix A for more information on support groups that might be in your area.)

In-Home Support

In many communities, in-home health care, personal care, and such homemaking services as cleaning, shopping, cooking, laundry, and minor home maintenance are available by contacting your county aging office or the county social services. There is usually a fee based on your ability to pay for in-home service.

Transportation

State aging services provide help for individuals age 60 and older who need specially adapted transportation. Specialized door-to-door transportation for persons whose disability limits independent mobility is available by contacting a local office on aging or one's county social services.

Medical Coverage

Medicare

Medicare is a federally funded health insurance program available to most people older than 65. Medicare has two parts of coverage — Part A, covering some hospital or skilled nursing facility inpatient care, and Part B, which covers doctor's services and certain types of out-patient care. Although one does pay a premium for the coverage that does not cover all your health care needs, it is an important benefit for people with high eye care costs. You are encouraged to apply for Medicare up to 3 months before turning 65. Even if you continue to work after age 65 and do not receive Social Security, you may be eligible for Medicare.

Medicaid

Medicaid is a federal/state health care program for people with limited income and resources. Although public health insurance covers both in-patient and out-patient medical eye care, guidelines vary by state. The health or social services office in your county can provide details.

Financial Assistance

Social Security, Supplemental Security Income (SSI), and food stamps are important resources for people with limited income. Most agencies can help you get eligibility information.

Social Security

Social Security is a federal program providing supplemental retirement income for a majority of people over age 65 (and for some beginning at age 62). Financial benefits may be available to the severely disabled, the retired worker and/or to his or her dependents, or to widows and widowers. Eligibility is not determined by your financial assets — you may have extensive savings, autos, or other property and still be eligible. Contact the nearest Social Security office as soon as, or even before, you feel you may be eligible. As a convenience to recipients, especially helpful for people with visual impairments not able to drive, direct deposit of your monthly benefit check to your local bank may be arranged.

Supplemental Security Income (SSI)

Supplemental Security Income (SSI) is a program often confused with Social Security. This is a joint federal/state program assuring a minimum level of income for people who are at least age 65, legally blind, or otherwise disabled. Unlike Social Security, you (and your spouse) must have limited financial resources to be eligible. Contact the nearest Social Security office to get more information or to apply.

Food Stamps

Food stamps are provided through a federal program to supplement the food buying ability of low-income individuals or families. Contact your county welfare or social services office.

Library Services

The U. S. National Library Service for the Blind and Physically Handicapped (NLS) of the Library of Congress provides reading materials to people who are unable to read standard print because of a physical or a mental condition. Books and magazines are available on cassette tape, on records, or in braille. These materials, as well as specially adapted machines required to hear tapes or records, are available for loan at no charge. Applications and eligibility information may be obtained from the state service for the blind or from your local library. See Chapter 17 for more information on library services.

Veterans' Benefits

Certain benefits may be available to veterans, their survivors, or to their parents with limited resources. The Department of Veterans Affairs has a network of rehabilitation centers and clinics that provide in-patient services to veterans who are legally blind or have low vision. Contact the local office of the Veterans Administration or your county veteran's service officer for details on the range of services.

Dog Guides

There are a number of schools in the United States wholly devoted to breeding, raising, and training dogs as mobility guides for blind persons. The schools typically require a student to stay at the facility for approximately 1 month. Because the training is rigorous, health factors are closely scrutinized on applications. At most schools, the charge for round-trip transportation, room and board, and training, as well as the dog, is on an ability to pay. If you are interested, but think you lack adequate financial resources, contact one of the schools in Appendix A for further information.

Health and Wellness Reassurance

The U. S. Postal Service's "Carrier Alert" program will notify a designated contact person if someone's mail is uncollected for 2 days. Contact your local carrier or the post office for details on this free service.

"Lifeline" type services are available in increasing numbers of communities for a monthly fee. An individual in distress can communicate with the local hospital via a necklace transmitter to summon emergency personnel.

Some community organizations offer a telephone reassurance program providing a daily call to a disabled or older person living alone. Contact your local aging office for information.

As was mentioned at the beginning of this chapter, coping with low vision should not be attempted without professional help. Although all of the preceding services can be helpful, each person with low vision will need to determine which resources can be most beneficial to help them cope with the loss of vision. Accepting rehabilitation or other supportive help is not a sign of weakness; it is a sign of strong determination to be as independent as you can.

Chapter 17

Common Questions and Concerns of People with Low Vision

Coping with low vision is an individual experience. No one else feels exactly like you do about it. But even though your experience is unique, people with low vision share many of the same daily problems and frustrations of living in a sighted world.

Following are some of the most common questions and concerns that people with low vision ask rehabilitation personnel. Because everyone's vision and personal circumstances are different, all of these strategies may not work for you. They are provided to help you become more aware that "something can, indeed, be done." Although many of the following approaches seem quite simple and obvious, you are urged to consult with a representative from your state's agency for the blind to ensure that the approach or strategy you choose is the best and safest for your personal circumstances.

Seeing Small Print

"I am now having difficulty seeing small print. If my eyes get worse as my doctor has informed me they might, how will I be able to read my mail, recipes, books, or the newspaper?"

Depending on your vision, you may find that magnifiers or closed-circuit televisions (CCTVs) will enable you to read standard print. Because each person's eyes are different, someone else's magnifier may work but is probably not the best one for you. Your eye doctor may be able to suggest a low vision clinic for a thorough evaluation to try out different types of optical and nonoptical aids. (See Chapter 12 for more on low vision aids.)

Talking Books

"I have a book on the history of Northeastern Wisconsin. As my great-grandparents and other relatives are mentioned in it, it has special significance to me. The print is now too small for me to read. Is there any way I can order it on Talking Books?"

The United States National Library Service for the Blind and Physically Handicapped (NLS) of the Library of Congress and the Canadian National Library for the Blind have free, specialized library services for patrons unable to read standard print. The Talking Book Program is a lending library of books and magazines on records or cassette tape or in braille. The library also loans, at no charge, the specially adapted cassette players and/or record players necessary to play these materials. The selection of books is extensive. Patrons may select such general categories of books as mysteries, romances, or westerns, or specific titles through the catalog listings sent periodically to readers.

Contact your local librarian or your state's agency for the blind for information and an application. This service is available to people who are unable to read standard print materials. People who are visually impaired may be eligible even if they benefit from the use of magnifiers.

Although the list of recorded materials is extensive, there isn't always the necessary demand for certain books to justify having them put into national circulation. Contact your Library for the Blind, local public library, or state services for the blind if you are interested in having a favorite book or any other print material transcribed onto cassette tape. In many communities, a local voluntary agency may provide this service. Because the recording is often done by volunteers, the only fee might be for the cost of the blank tapes.

Religious Materials

"I was told by a friend that the Library for the Blind has only a limited number of copies of the Bible available to lend. Is there any place I could buy a copy of the Bible on cassette tape?"

Specialized religious materials such as scriptures are available on cassette tape from certain organizations. (See Appendix A.) Many larger book stores now sell a wide variety of books on cassette tape. The Library for the Blind has listings of many religious documents available on tape or in large print. The administrative office of the particular religion may have information on the availability of specific materials.

Handwriting

"Now that my vision has decreased, I am having a hard time staying on the line when I sign my name or write letters. My children say they can always read my letters, but I'd still like my writing to look neat. Is there anything that would help?"

Instruction from a rehabilitation teacher on the proper use of signature and writing guides can make accomplishment of these daily living skills almost routine. Many people find that bold point pens and markers make it much easier to see where and what they have written. One of the simplest and most effective products is a pad of stationery with very bold, widely spaced lines to enhance writing ease. Simple signature guides are pieces of plastic the size of a credit card with a signature-size window cut into them (see illustration on this page).

Script-writing templates for writing letters, grocery lists, and phone directories, are made of black plastic or cardboard to enable staying on the line almost automatically

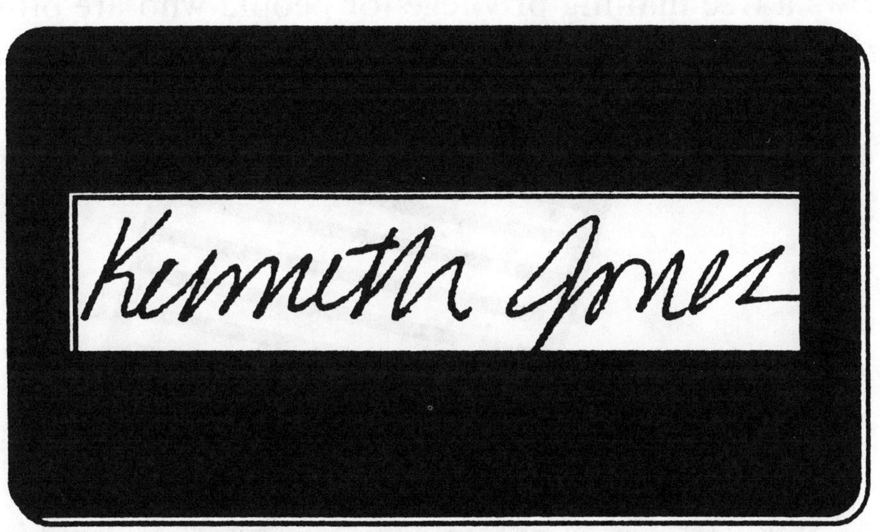

A credit-card size black plastic guide is helpful for signing your name.

(see illustration on this page). Other guides, with strings, metal, or black plastic frames mounted on a clipboard are also available.

Free Mailing Privilege

"My sister, who also has age-related maculopathy, lives in a different state. We both have very limited incomes so we can't talk on the phone very often. Because we have to write so large, even a short letter requires three postage stamps. Is there any service available to help us afford the postage we use?"

The United States Congress recognized this need and allows a free mailing privilege for people who are blind

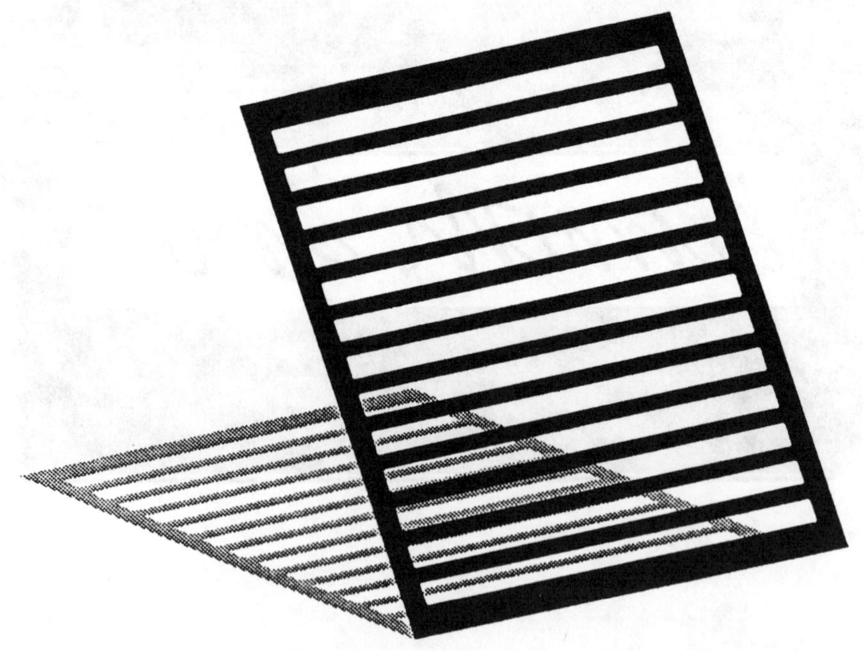

A black plastic script writing template makes staying on the line automatic when writing letters on plain paper.

or who cannot use or read conventional print material due to a physical handicap (see illustration on this page). Because the increased weight of braille, large print, and recordings increases postage cost, the law allows such matter to be mailed for free. To qualify, your doctor or another competent professional must certify that you are unable to read standard reading material. You must file this statement at your local post office.

There are some restrictions; for instance, the envelope must be left unsealed to allow postal inspection and no advertising is allowed. The words "Free Matter for the Blind or Handicapped" must appear in place of the stamp. Rubber stamps or preprinted stickers of this statement are conveniently available from some consumer products catalogs. Talk to your mail carrier or ask at the local post office for the brochure that explains details.

The words, "Free Matter For The Blind," **in place of the stamp allow large print, cassette tape, or braille letters to be sent postage-free.**

Many people now mail "voice" letters on cassette tapes. Specially designed mailing containers are available that hold up to four tapes. Most have a window for a double-sided label. One side of the label has "From:" you, and "To:" your recipient, and the opposite side reverses the names. You simply listen to the taped letter, record your reply letter, flip the label to the other side, and put in the mailbox. See one of the consumer products catalogs (Appendix A) for mailer sources or contact your state's agency for the blind. Eligible persons may send taped letters as "Free Matter for the Blind."

Money Handling

"I am having a great deal of difficulty finding the correct change at the grocery check-out counter and in identifying quarters for the laundry equipment in my apartment complex. Is there an easy way for me to tell a nickel from a quarter, or a one dollar bill from a ten?"

Coins may be identified by feeling the edges with your thumbnail. The two least valuable coins, the penny and the nickel, both have smooth, unfinished edges, with the dime and quarter both having a milled edge that feels like a series of ridges. The size differences between each type of coin makes correct identification quite foolproof (see illustration on the facing page).

Coin purses with separate channels for each size coin are a helpful way of organizing change. Some people with visual impairments use a 35 mm film canister or a simi-

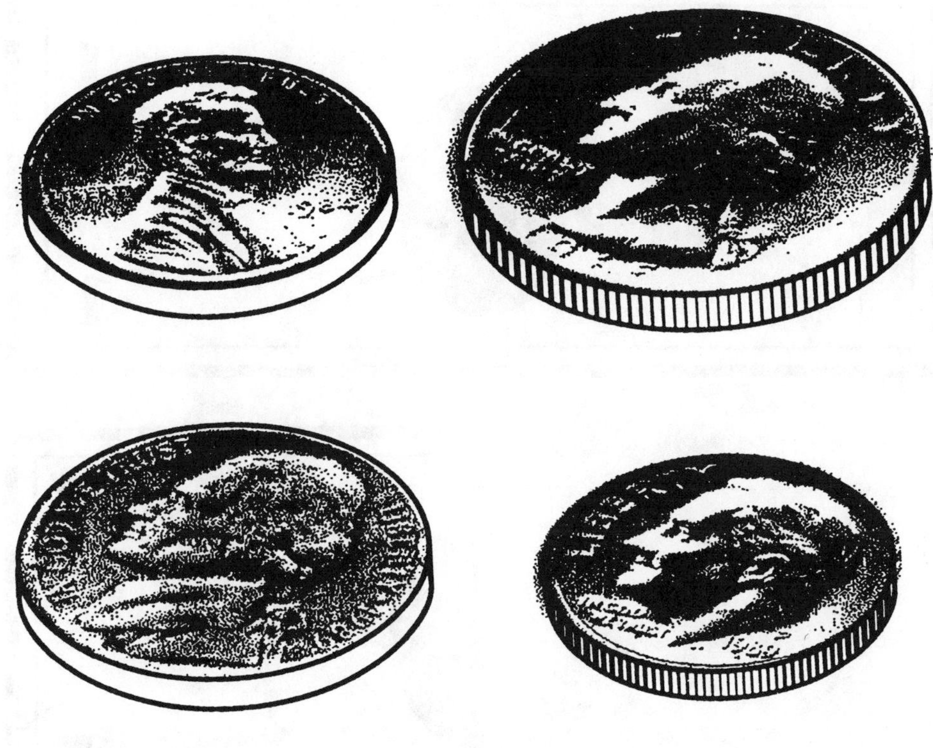

Notice the smooth or milled edges of the different coins.

larly sized prescription bottle to keep quarters for their laundromat trips.

Many people with low vision keep their paper money organized by folding the different denominations in various ways (see illustration on page 134). You might try leaving your one dollar bills unfolded, the fives may be folded in half so they are almost a square, the tens might be folded in half the long way, and a twenty can be folded like a ten dollar bill and then folded over a second time. Another common way to handle money is to put the different bills in different compartments of your wallet.

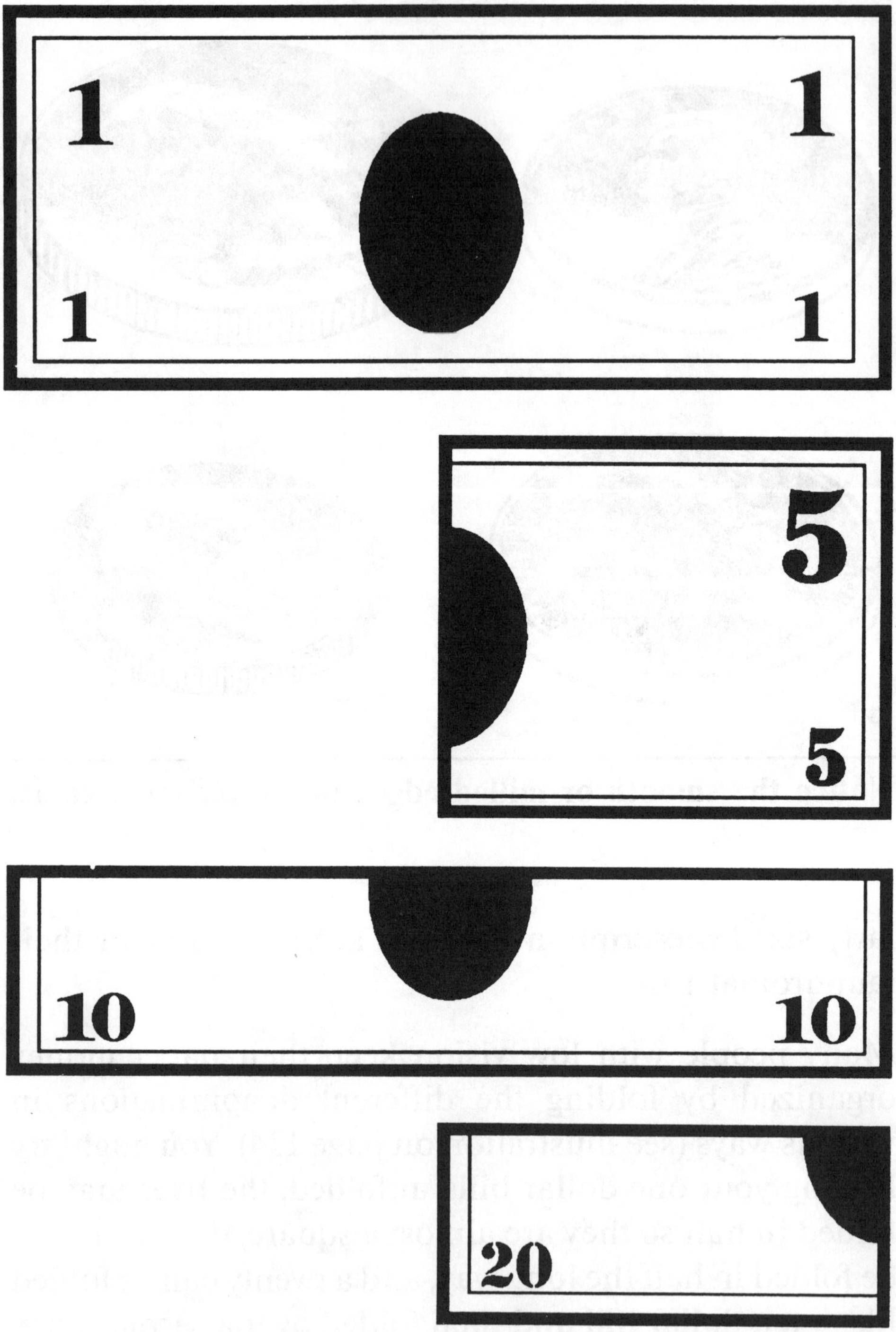

This suggested method for folding paper money makes identification easy.

Still another method to simplify the identification of bills is to limit your paper money to just ones and fives and keep them in separate compartments or pockets.

Dials and Thermostats

"I am having trouble setting the correct temperatures on my household thermostat and oven. It seems so dark that I try using a flashlight. This doesn't always help me enough to be sure. Is there anything to help me?"

A permanent magic marker may be used to enlarge a temperature setting mark on many appliances or dials (see illustration on this page). A well-placed, goose-neck

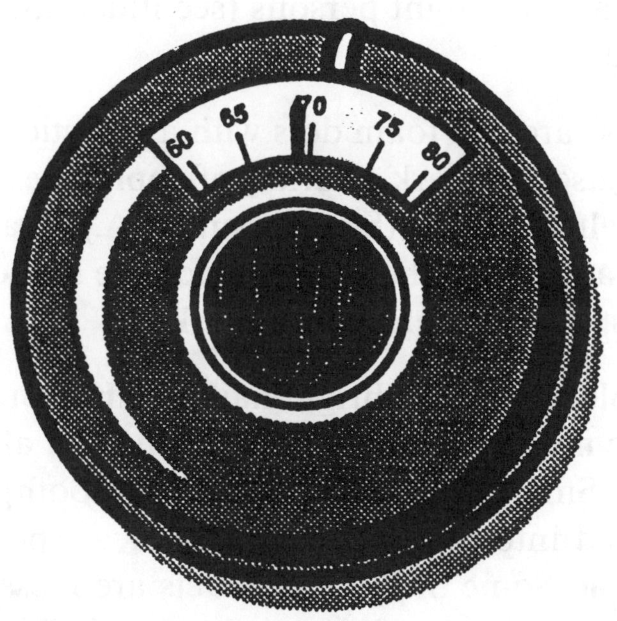

A household thermostat can be marked with very dark, bold lines.

lamp or a flashlight may be all that's needed to make the dial visible.

When extra lighting isn't sufficient, other useful products might do the trick. "HiMarks" is a bright orange paint-like material that comes in a tube like toothpaste. (See Consumer Products in Appendix A.) This material is used to put thin lines or dots at the desired settings on various household items, including laundry equipment, tools, measuring cups or spoons, rulers, stoves, microwave ovens, radios, and televisions. When dry, the marks are both easy to see and feel.

Another marking product, called "LocDots," has self-adhesive, raised dots on a clear plastic filmstrip. These are especially helpful for marking typewriter and computer keyboards, dials, or other devices that must also be seen by average-sight persons (see illustration on the facing page).

"TouchDots" are soft foam dots with a self-stick backing that can be used to mark a variety of appliances, tools, or other household items. (See Appendix A.) Available in both white and black, they can provide the highest possible contrast on the item being marked.

Many people simply use bright nail polish to put a small mark at the most commonly used settings on all of their appliances. Small beads or sections of a toothpick may also be glued into place using epoxy or a type of super glue. **Caution:** Some of these products are messy at best and may be dangerous if not used properly. If in doubt, get assistance or magnify product instructions to follow carefully package directions.

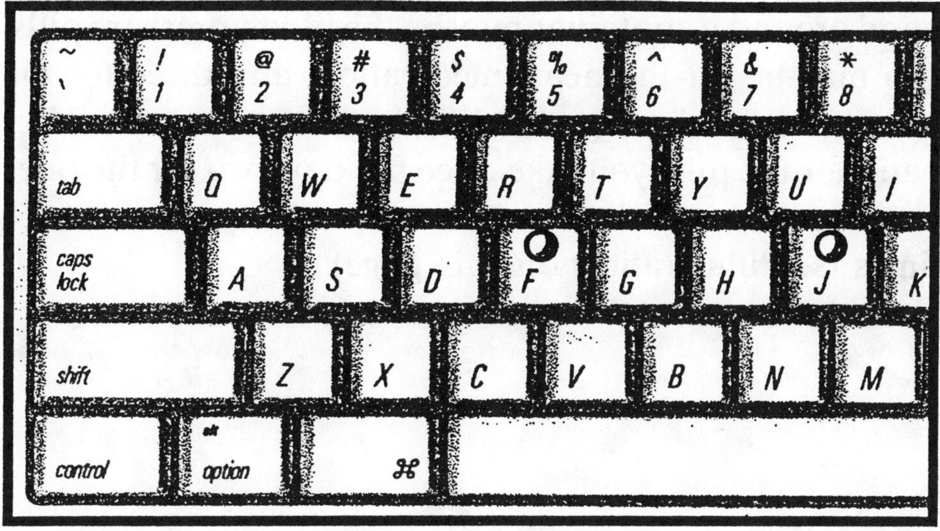

The keys on a typewriter or a computer can be much easier to locate following application of raised dots.

Prescriptions

"My mother is now taking five different prescriptions, some appearing quite similar. How can she be sure she is taking the right medicine at the right time?"

Sometimes, problems with the identification of prescription medications can be avoided at the time of purchase. Simply request a different shape for each medicine or even oversized containers to differentiate between your medicines. If no children are likely to have access to your medicines, you may request other than "child proof" lids.

Some people with visual impairments use a rubber band code for each type of medication or for the number of times it is to be taken per day. For instance, one rubber band around a container may be the blood pressure pills, two may be for the heart medication, and three for the pain pills. Another approach would be to use one rubber band for the pills you take once per day, two for the ones you take twice per day, and three for those you take three times (see illustration on this page).

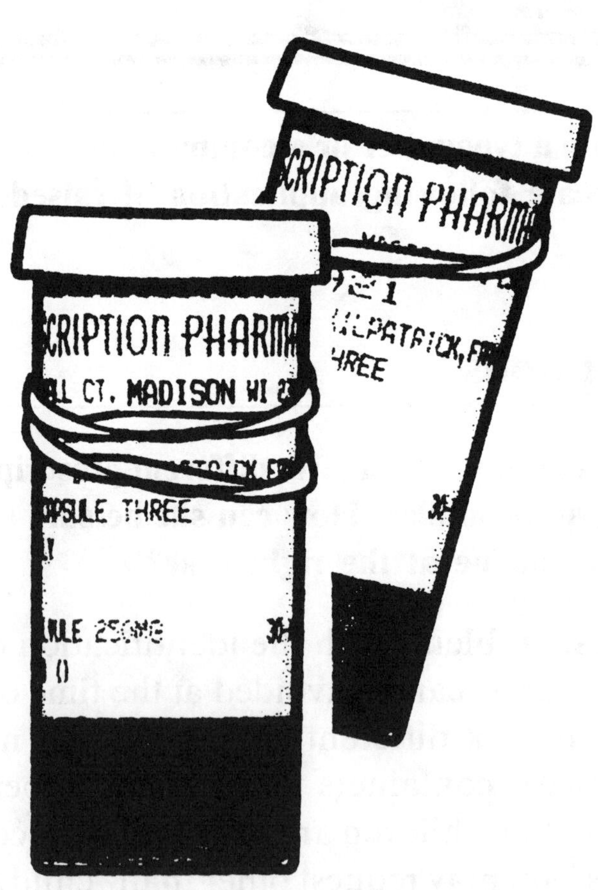

Notice how prescription bottles may be plainly marked with rubber bands to simplify identification.

A handy product is a 7-day pillbox with four separate lidded compartments for each day (see illustration on this page). Each lid is labeled "Morning," "Noon," "Evening," or "Bedtime" so it is quite easy to take and to verify that you have already taken the proper medications. (See Consumer Products in Appendix A.)

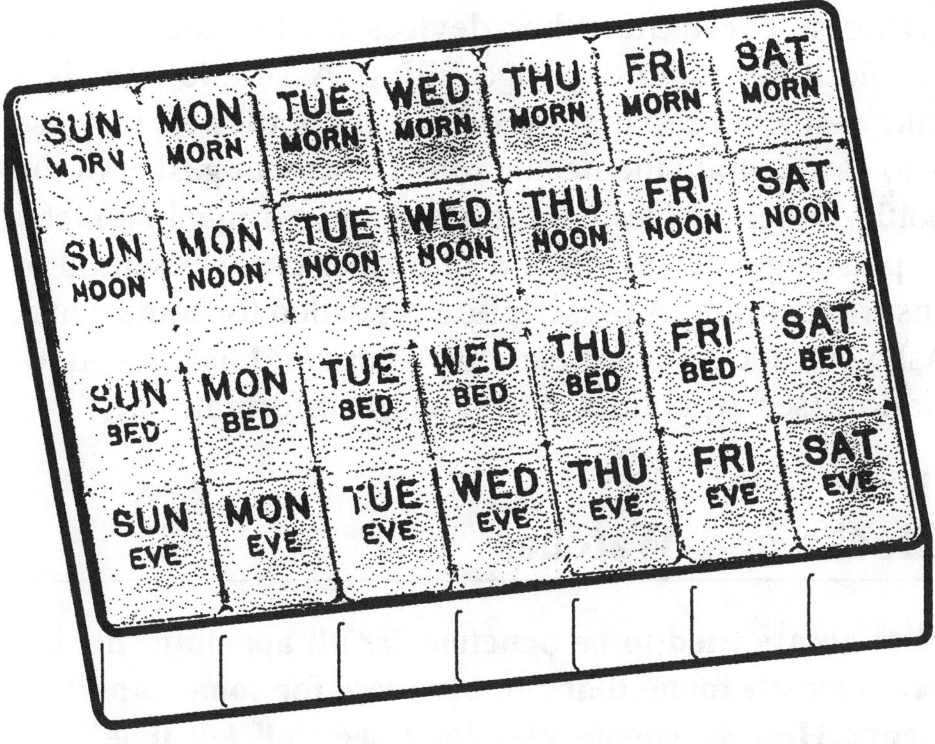

A 7-day plastic pillbox with four compartments for each day and "Morn," "Noon," "Eve," and "Bed" can be helpful.

Diabetes Management

"It's getting more difficult to see well enough to accurately fill my own insulin syringes. Even though I feel I could give my own injections with my eyes closed, I'm very concerned that I get the proper dose of insulin. What do other people with diabetes do?"

It really depends on the individual. If you don't fully trust your vision *all the time,* you may try getting assistance to accurately fill a supply of syringes. Some people benefit from a low-power, clip-on magnifier made for insulin syringes. There are other devices on the market that enable independent syringe filling. A simple item is a funnel-shaped cap that fits on insulin bottles. Its purpose is to easily guide the needle into the rubber gasket of the bottle. Other devices hold the vial and syringe in a metal or plastic guide. Instruction in proper use is essential to ensure accuracy. A prescription is needed for some items. Ask your doctor or contact the American Diabetes Association (see Appendix A) for more information.

Clocks and Watches

"I've always tried to be punctual for all appointments but have recently found that I've been late for some important events. How do people who can't see well tell time?"

Large-print, talking, and tactile clocks and watches (see illustration on page 141) are all available through the various consumer products catalog companies listed in Appendix A. A few cautions: The "voice" quality of some

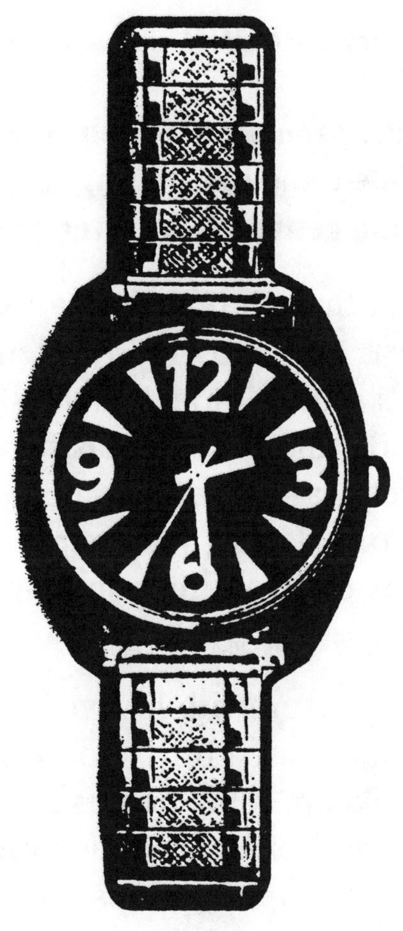

A large-print wristwatch with only 12, 3, 6, and 9 marked.

talking devices is very high pitched and may be difficult for some people to hear clearly. Also, the procedure for resetting the time when batteries have been replaced or at "daylight" time changes is very complicated on some watches. Large print is interpreted differently by various manufacturers and not all raised markings are easy to feel. If at all possible, arrange for a trial of different timepieces with a rehabilitation teacher prior to purchasing one.

Shaving and Applying Makeup

"How can I handle grooming like shaving, applying makeup, or even a simple thing like getting the toothpaste on the toothbrush without getting it all over me also?"

Some people find that changing to an electric shaver is the easiest, safest, and most convenient way to shave. Unless a person's sense of touch is very poor, it is usually easy to locate the unshaved areas by feel. If you've always used a safety razor, you should be encouraged to continue to use one. Using your sense of touch to find the slippery areas of remaining shaving cream is a key to remember.

A useful aid for a person with low vision is a magnifying mirror to enhance your ability to verify your desired application of makeup. A big help is having a friend provide immediate and honest feedback on how well it has been applied. Some support groups for people with visual impairments sponsor workshops covering the proper application of makeup.

A trick some people use is to simply squeeze toothpaste onto their index finger first and then transfer it to the brush or to their mouth. Those who live alone or have their own separate tubes may simply squeeze toothpaste directly into their mouths.

Housecleaning Patterns

"How will I be able to do my own cleaning?"

Organization of both supplies and approach is the key to successful cleaning. Virtually any surface to be cleaned may be mentally divided into a grid-like pattern. For example, the recommended approach to clean a rectangular tabletop is to wipe on a straight path down one edge, move your hand over almost the width of the sponge or cloth, and go back up along the previous line. Continue this up and back overlapping pattern across the entire surface. After you've finished, move to the next closest side of the table and repeat the pattern. By cleaning the surface twice and at right angles, you are virtually assured that the entire surface will be adequately covered.

Shopping

"How can I more easily handle my own shopping?"

Shopping presents a special challenge. Some people make arrangements with the store manager to receive an escort. Choosing hours and days when the store is least busy usually makes such special requests for assistance easier for merchants to respond to. Others go with a friend. You may find that using an optical aid or magnifier to more easily read labels may make it convenient to verify the contents of similarly packaged items. In many communities, low- or no-cost delivery is also available.

Helpers might try using rubber bands to attach large-print labels on canned goods as you shop or when you unpack groceries at home (see illustration on page 144). When the item is used, the label goes into the "shopping

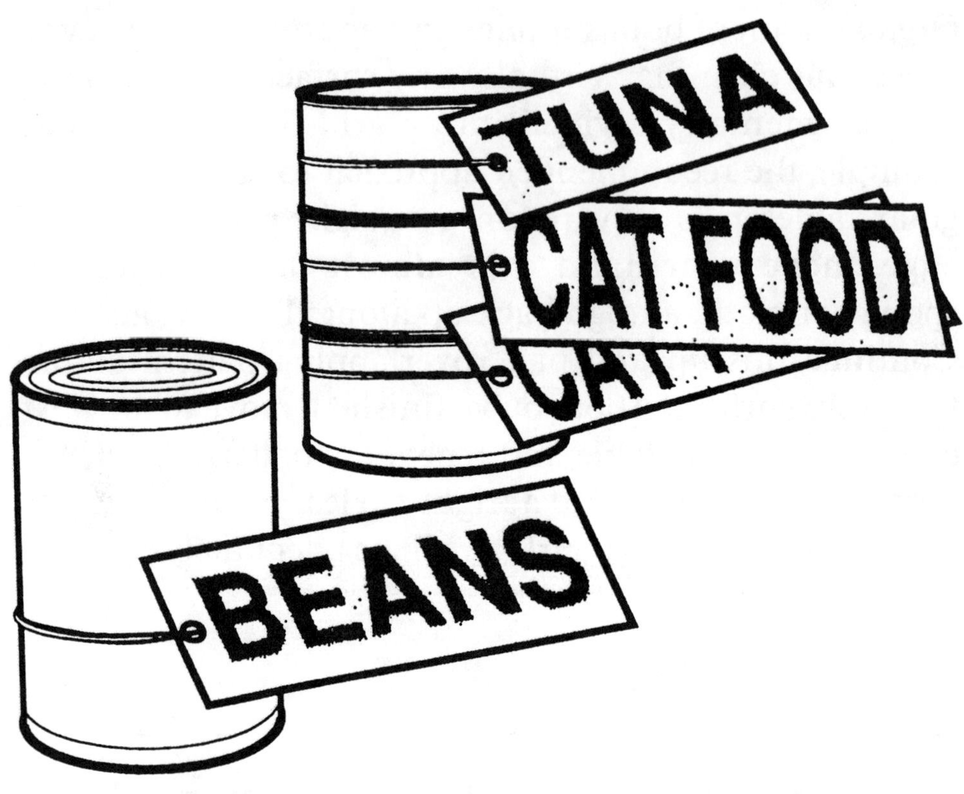

Large print labels with rubber bands for attaching to canned goods. Foods labeled "BEANS," "TUNA," and "CAT FOOD" are much easier to identify.

list" envelope and is transferred to the new item at the store or as soon as possible after returning home.

Cooking

"How can I safely prepare my own meals?

Many people, especially those who live alone, find that a microwave is the ideal kitchen appliance. Because microwave ovens cook quickly yet stay cool, they are perfect for the safe heating or reheating of many foods. A wide variety of new convenient microwaveable foods continue to be introduced.

Direct instruction from a rehabilitation teacher is recommended prior to the resumption of unfamiliar tasks. Many catalog suppliers have items that have been adapted to make food preparation much easier. These include large-print, raised-print, or braille timers (see illustration on this page); large-print and cassette-recorded cookbooks; measuring spoons and cups with large-print or tactile markings; slicing guides allowing safe and uniform slicing of meats, breads, and vegetables; oven mitts; and a large variety of labeling and marking products.

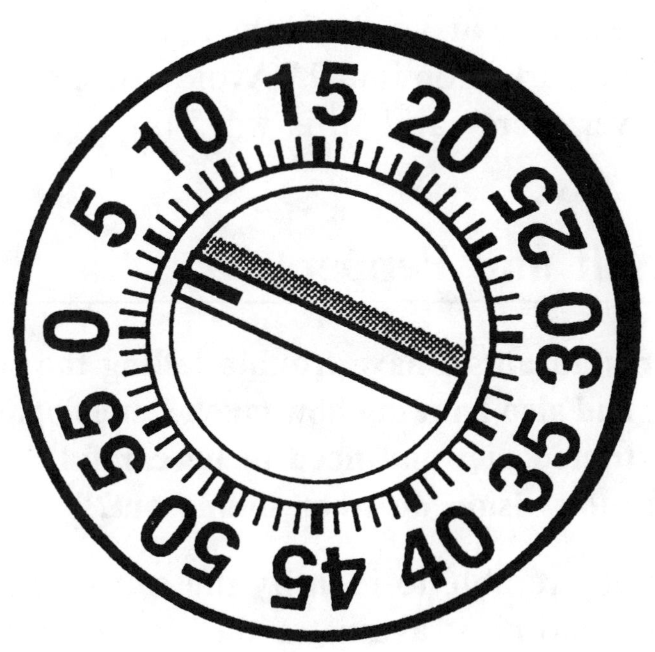

A large print kitchen timer.

Elbow-length oven mitts offer the highest degree of safety for handling hot utensils.

Identifying Food on a Plate

"Because of her poor eyesight, my wife and I recently stopped going to the local senior citizens center for the noon meal. We'd like to continue going, because we have many good friends who always go. How can I help my wife identify the food on her plate or locate the items on the table?"

A common strategy is to use the "face of a clock" method (see illustration on page 147). Indicating that the salt and pepper is at 10 o'clock, the water glass is at 2, and the butter is at 6 will make locating objects much easier. Use the same directions for items on the plate. You might try saying, "The beans are at 3 o'clock, the mashed potatoes are at 12, and the pork chop is at 9." Avoid nonspecific terms such as "over there" and "this way."

Using Salt and Pepper

"In dark restaurants I have trouble telling the salt from the pepper and also knowing how much I'm using. I'm on a sodium-restricted diet and need to be careful. What can people with low vision do when dining out?"

Some people are able to identify the salt in clear glass shakers by holding it against a dark background. The light color then shows up. A number of points to remember: given equal amounts, salt is much heavier than

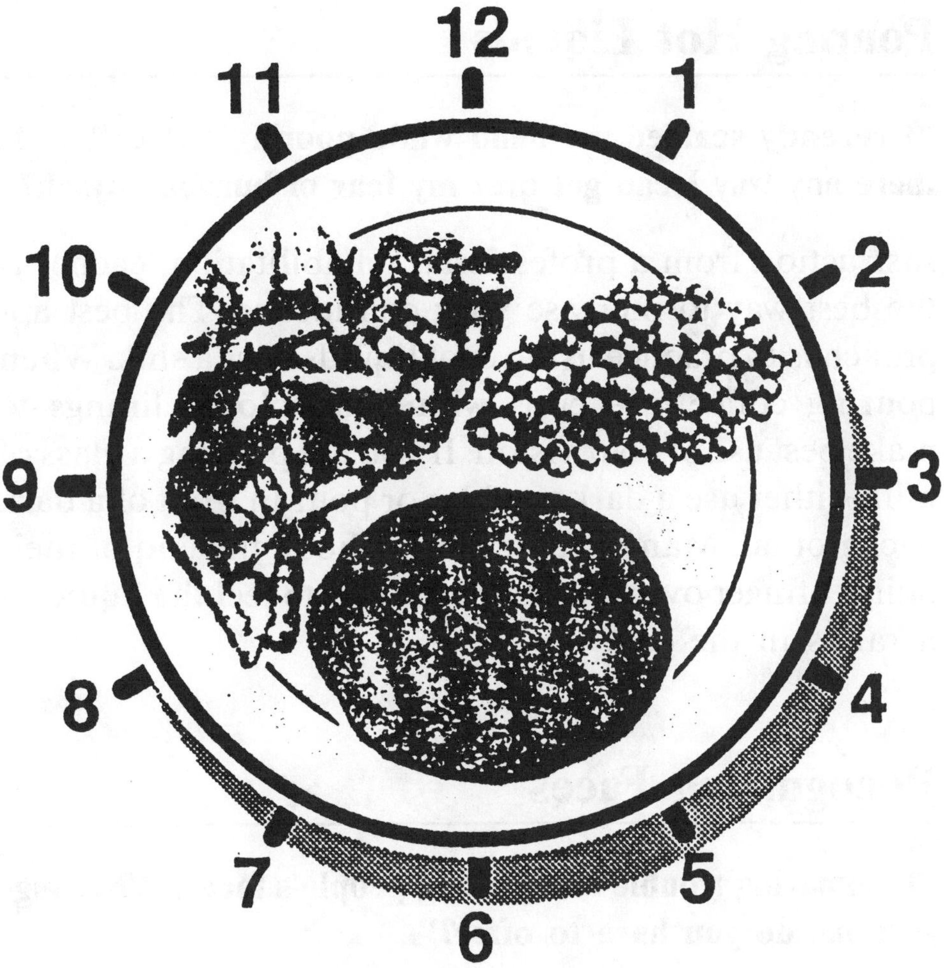

Items on a plate of food can be located if a friend uses the "face of a clock" method to orient you.

pepper, the top will be more slippery on the pepper shaker, and the smell is a sure sign. Try sprinkling some into the palm of your hand to feel the gritty texture of salt from the powdery feel of pepper.

To control the amount of salt you use, simply sprinkle some through your spread-out fingers held over your food.

Pouring Hot Liquids

"I recently scalded my hand while pouring hot coffee. Is there any way I can get over my fear of burning myself?"

Instruction from a professional rehabilitation teacher is the best way to increase your confidence. The best approach is to practice using cool liquids over a sink. When pouring coffee, use cups with light-colored linings to make best use of your vision. If you are pouring a glass of milk, either use a dark tumbler or pour in front of a dark background. Many people simply hook the end of their pointer finger over the rim of the cup to feel the liquid as it raises in the cup.

Recognizing Faces

"I am having trouble recognizing people's faces. What suggestions do you have to offer?"

Difficulty recognizing people's faces is one of the most common concerns of people who have visual impairments. You should begin informing friends that you are having this difficulty and that it would be helpful for them to announce their name when you meet. With practice, you may find that you are able to use your other senses more effectively. For instance, your sense of hearing can help you estimate a person's height by knowing where the voice is coming from. Your sense of touch can easily distinguish between a rough, calloused handshake and one that is soft. Some people may be identified by the smell of a distinctive cologne or perfume.

If you have a central vision loss such as maculopathy, you might try using your eccentric (or side) vision for best vision. You can try to look to the side when you need to see a friend's face. (There is more on eccentric vision in Chapter 13.)

Using "Look" and "See"

"I've been trying to avoid words like "look" and "see" around my father since he became legally blind. What are the accepted substitutes blind people feel comfortable with?"

You shouldn't try to avoid the use of "look" or "see," as the words are a standard part of our everyday language and there are really no good substitutes. Besides, blind people use "look" and "see" just as often as anyone else.

Color Contrast

"Since my eye condition came on, I've had a hard time seeing countertop edges, pot handles, serving containers at the table, the edge of the coffee table, and generally seeing small items in poor light. Do you have any suggestions?"

Most people with low vision find that black (or a very dark solid color) against a white (or very light background) is the easiest to see. Avoiding use of floral pattern and plaid tablecloths will help you locate small items on a table more easily.

Some people who enjoy working on crafts use a cafeteria-style tray with half of it covered with contrasting contact paper. This half-light and half-dark arrangement will allow you to more easily find dark items on the light side and vice versa.

A strip of black plastic electrical tape on a light counter edge will help when moving items in the kitchen from refrigerator or cupboard. Be creative! Use strips of white plastic tape on black pot handles and put white or light-colored books near the edge of a dark coffee table.

Bright Sunlight

"I am having a difficult time adjusting to either very bright or very dim light. Will regular sunglasses help?"

As we age, most of us develop photophobia — an increased sensitivity to bright sunlight. Sunglasses that filter the infrared and ultraviolet light have been found to relieve the irritation. See your eye doctor or low vision therapist for further information and check with your eye doctor to rule out other problems.

Receiving Help

"The medication I am taking is a diuretic that causes frequent urination. Because of my poor vision, I am very self-conscious about getting lost when I go into public restrooms. I recently became quite embarrassed when I unsuccessfully tried to open the wrong door. No one told me I was trying to open the door to the maintenance closet. How can I avoid this embarrassment so I can continue to make shopping trips to the mall?"

Even though their vision may be good enough to see steps, curbs, or other ground-level obstructions, many people who are legally blind carry a white cane for identification purposes. Because a white cane is a nearly universally accepted sign of blindness, someone is likely to offer needed assistance. Contact your state's agency for the blind to see if you meet the legal requirement to carry a white cane.

Travel

"For safety reasons, I gave up my license and no longer drive. I do love to travel but have found I need some form of picture identification to cash checks. I know I couldn't pass the driver's license eye test but I'd like to see about getting my old identification back. Is this possible?"

Some states offer a "Non Valid Driver's License" or state photo ID card for people who, for various reasons, don't drive. Contact the driver's license or motor vehicle office nearest you for availability and details. There will be a cost.

The American Foundation for the Blind in New York offers a picture identification card for people who are legally blind. In addition to the identification value, it may also help you qualify for a discount for certain bus fares or other services. See Appendix A for the listing for The American Foundation for the Blind for more information. Some municipalities offer disability photo identification services.

Support Groups

"Since my condition worsened as a result of a rare condition called maculopathy, I've started feeling quite isolated. Are there any organizations that offer a place to meet for people like me?"

First, you are definitely not alone in having maculopathy and you may find a great deal of support meeting others who also have it. Developing support groups for people with all types of visual impairments has become common for many rehabilitation service agencies. It is realized that peer support and the resultant sharing that emerges is extremely important for people as they adjust to living with low vision.

The purposes of peer support groups may include:

1. To establish a network in the community between people with visual impairments, family members and friends, and services and programs available for their support.

2. To provide a regular meeting place where people with visual impairments may meet, have dinner, and enjoy fellowship.

3. To provide information about programs and services available at the local, state, and national level for people with visual impairments and concerned others.

4. To raise community awareness of the special needs of people with visual impairments.

5. To advocate for the well-being of people with visual impairments.
6. To provide opportunities for people with visual impairments and concerned others to participate in community activities.
7. To establish programs/services that enhance the dignity and independence of people with visual impairments.
8. To allow people with visual impairments to be volunteers in senior centers and the community.

Often people are unaware of support groups that would benefit those who are blind or who have visual impairments as well as friends, family members, and significant others who may wish to be included.

Support groups for people with low vision may meet at senior citizen centers, nutrition sites, senior citizen apartment complexes, local restaurants or cafes, service club meeting spaces, or private residences. Contact your state's services for the blind for further information.

Something Can Be Done

The preceding strategies are merely a select few developed, invented, and refined by rehabilitation personnel and people with visual impairments. We hope the hints will help you better cope with the everyday frustrations of low vision. The strategies demonstrate that solutions are available for overcoming the challenges you face. The hints are not intended to replace the direct instruction from rehabilitation professionals who can personalize their help to your individual needs.

For more information on specialized products or services for people with visual impairments, contact your state's services for the blind or see "Consumer Products" in Appendix A.

Appendix A

Resources to Cope with Low Vision

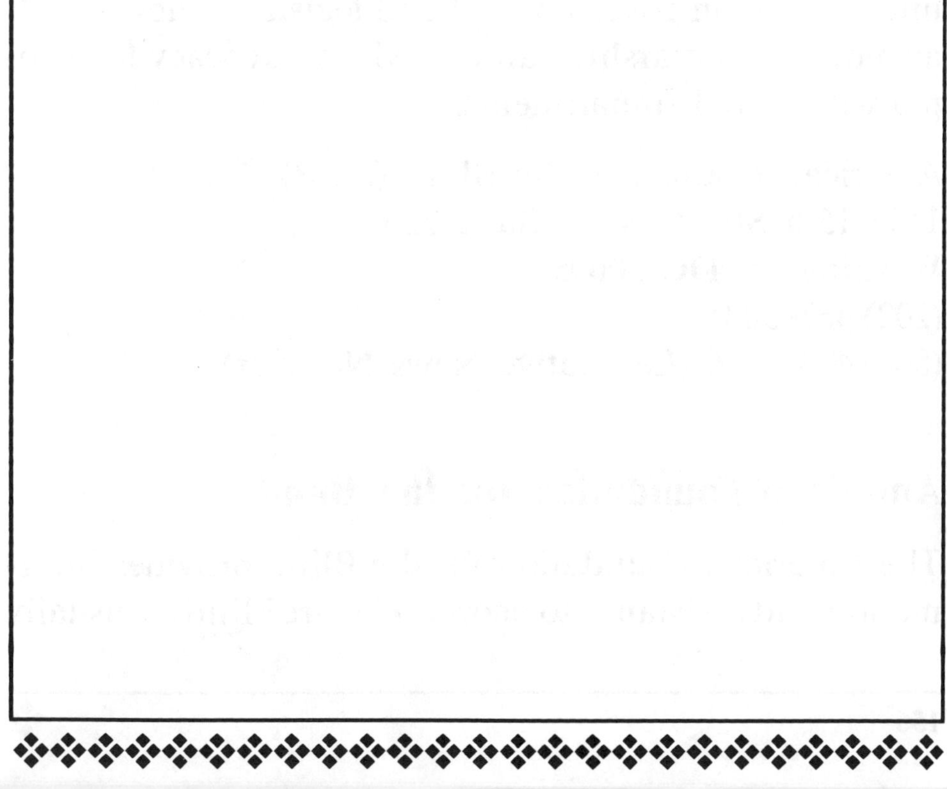

The following organizations provide a wide range of supportive services for people with limited vision. Many have a toll-free 800 number for your use. Although most of the following have no fixed limits on the geographical service area, you may be referred to a resource near you or to a local affiliate, if applicable. There may be charges for the services offered, so please ask before you order anything.

National Consumer and Advocacy Organizations

American Council of the Blind (ACB)

ACB publishes *The Braille Forum,* a magazine in large type, cassette tape, and in braille on issues of interest to people with low vision or blindness. They also offer a "Washington Connection" toll-free number for current information on governmental and legislative news. ACB also offers scholarships and provides advocacy for people with visual impairments.

American Council of the Blind (ACB)
1155 15th Street, N.W., Suite 720
Washington, DC 20005
(202) 467–5081
(800) 424–8666 (Legislative News Number)

American Foundation for the Blind

The American Foundation for the Blind provides information and assistance to people who are blind or visually impaired, their families, and professionals serving their needs. Vision loss issue books and other materials are published in braille and on cassette tape. The foundation records and produces talking books on disk and cassette tape, as well as producing and selling specially adapted consumer products. A library on literature about blindness is maintained.

American Foundation for the Blind
15 West 16th Street
New York, NY 10011
(800) 232-5463
(212) 620-2000

Association for Education and Rehabilitation of the Blind and Visually Impaired (AERBVI)

AERBVI is the international membership association of professionals interested in the promotion, development, and improvement of all phases of education and rehabilitation of blind and visually impaired children and adults. This organization represents professionals in the fields of education of children or the rehabilitation of adults who are blind or are visually impaired.

Association for Education and Rehabilitation
of the Blind and Visually Impaired
206 North Washington Street
Suite 320
Alexandria, VA 22314
(703) 548-1884

Association for Macular Diseases, Inc.

This not-for-profit member organization advocates on behalf of individuals with conditions affecting the macula. The group promotes education and research on the causes of macular degeneration and other conditions. This organization is a support group and clearinghouse for information and referral for people who have macular diseases.

Association for Macular Diseases, Inc.
210 East 64th Street
New York, NY 10021
(212) 605-3719

Council of Citizens with Low Vision

This not-for-profit organization advocates on behalf of people with low vision, provides information and referral services, sponsors seminars and conferences on low vision, provides scholarships to students in vision rehabilitation programs, and publishes a quarterly newsletter, *The CCLV News.* Public education is provided.

Council of Citizens with Low Vision
Riley Tower 2, Suite 2300
600 North Alabama Street
Indianapolis, IN 46204-1415
(317) 638-8822
(800) 733-2258

Helen Keller National Center

Serves deaf-blind adults through its national, regional, and local affiliates. Provides technical assistance and training on issues of both hearing and vision loss.

Helen Keller National Center
111 Middle Neck Road
Sands Point, NY 11050-1299
(516) 944-8900
FAX (516) 944-7302

Lions Clubs International

The Lions Clubs International have numerous local clubs. The motto of Lions is "We Serve." The main mission of Lions has been to provide a wide range of support to people who are blind, have visual impairments, or who are otherwise disabled.

Lions Clubs International
300 22nd Street
Oak Brook, IL 60570
(312) 571-5466

National Accreditation Council

The National Accreditation Council (NAC) is dedicated to the improvement of services for people who are blind or visually impaired. NAC establishes a professional team who volunteer to conduct onsite reviews of agencies. The standards they follow have been developed by professionals and agencies and are open to comment and revision.

National Accreditation Council
232 Madison Avenue, Suite 907
New York, NY 10016
(212) 779-8080

National Association for the Visually Handicapped (NAVH)

NAVH is a nonprofit, national organization solely devoted to the partially seeing. The group provides unique programs of practical and emotional support for people of all ages. Free, large-print newsletters and a "Visual Aids and Informational Material" catalog are published. Services are provided free, so that impaired vision need not mean impaired life. Information and referrals to resources in your area are provided.

National Association for the
Visually Handicapped (NAVH)
22 West 21st Street
New York, NY 10010
(212) 889-3141

(On the West Coast)

NAVH
3201 Balboa Street
San Francisco, CA 94121
(415) 221-3201

National Federation of the Blind (NFB)

NFB is an advocacy organization providing a variety of support programs for people who are blind or visually impaired. Scholarships, a speakers bureau, and publications are available. Affiliates operate throughout the United States.

National Federation of the Blind (NFB)
1800 Johnson Street
Baltimore, MD 21230
(301) 659-9314

Consumer Products

The following organizations offer free catalogs listing a wide range of adaptive equipment for sale. The items they sell have been found to be useful for people with low vision.

Aids Unlimited
1101 North Calvert Street
Baltimore, MD 21202
(410) 659-0232

American Foundation for the Blind
Consumer Products
15 West 16th Street
New York, NY 10011
(201) 862-8838

American Printing House for the Blind
1839 Frankfort Avenue
Louisville, KY 40206
(502) 895–2405

Diabetes Supplies
8181 North Stadium Drive
Houston, TX 77054-1826
(713) 622–5587
(800) 622–5587

Howe Press
Perkins School for the Blind
175 North Beacon Street
Watertown, MA 02172
(617) 924–3434

Independent Living Aids, Inc.
27 East Mall
Plainview, NY 11803
(800) 537–2118

Maxi Aids
42 Executive Boulevard
P.O. Box 3209
Farmingdale, NY 11735
(800) 522–6294

Science Products for the Blind
P.O. Box 888
Southeastern, PA 19399
(800) 888–7400

TeleSensory
455 North Bernardo Avenue
Mountain View, CA 94043
(415) 960-0920
(800) 227-8418
FAX (415) 969-9064

The Lighthouse
Low Vision Products
36-02 Northern Boulevard
Long Island City, NY 11101
(800) 453-4923
(718) 937-9338

L. S. & S. Group, Inc.
P.O. Box 673
Northbrook, IL 60065
(800) 468-4789
(708) 498-9777 (in Illinois)
FAX (708) 498-1482

Vis Aids
10209 Jamaica Avenue
P.O. Box 26
Richmond Hill, NY 11418
(800) 346-9579
(718) 847-4734
FAX (718) 441-2550

Dog Guides

The following organizations may be contacted for information about the acquisition and use of a dog guide. Each school has its own eligibility policies and costs. You can expect to be asked to provide a statement from your doctor verifying your physical condition and your ability to walk at a vigorous pace. Some groups may require a referral from a rehabilitation professional from a recognized agency serving people who are blind or visually impaired.

The Seeing Eye, Inc.
P.O. Box 375
Morristown, NJ 07960
(201) 539-4425

Guide Dog Foundation for the Blind
371 East Jericho Turnpike
Smithtown, NY 11787
(800) 548-4337

Leader Dogs for the Blind
1039 Rochester Road
Rochester, MI 48307
(313) 651-9011

Guide Dogs for the Blind, Inc.
P.O. Box 151200
San Rafael, CA 94915-1200
(415) 499-4000
FAX (415) 499-4035

Guiding Eyes for the Blind
611 Granite Springs Road
Yorktown Heights, NY 10598
(914) 245-4024

Health-Enhancing Organizations

The organizations listed below provide health enhancing services for people who may be older, have visual impairments, or related concerns.

American Diabetes Association

The American Diabetes Association provides educational services related to diabetes and health concerns related to diabetes. Local affiliates are listed in the white pages of your telephone directory. For American Diabetes Association membership information and a free, 1-year subscription to their quarterly newsletter, call 1-800-232-3472.

American Diabetes Association
1660 Duke Street
Alexandria, VA 22314
(703) 549-1500
(800) 232-3472

Foundation for Glaucoma Research

This national organization is committed to protecting the sight of people with glaucoma through research and education. Members receive a quarterly newsletter, GLEAMS. The group is devoted to research, developing support networks, and conducting studies related to glaucoma.

Foundation for Glaucoma Research
Suite 830
490 Post Street
San Francisco, CA 94102-1409
(414) 986–3162

National Eye Care Project

This national project provides free eye examinations, and possibly treatment, for older people who have limited financial resources *and* who do not have medical coverage.

National Eye Care Project
P.O. Box 9688
San Francisco, CA 94101-9688
(800) 222–EYES (222–3937)

Retinitis Pigmentosa (RP) Foundation Fighting Blindness

This organization provides information and referral to those interested in services, support networks, and physician referrals. The main focus of the foundation is to provide funds for research into the cause and cure of RP and related retinal degenerations. Contact the national office for the nearest local affiliate.

Retinitis Pigmentosa (RP) Foundation
Fighting Blindness
1401 Mount Royal Avenue
4th Floor
Baltimore, MD 21217
(800) 683-5555 Toll Free
(410) 255-9400
(410) 225-9409 TDD

National Society to Prevent Blindness

This is a national organization with many state affiliates whose mission is to prevent blindness through visual screening. The organization conducts public education on eye hazards and industrial safety, and has publications and videos available on various eye conditions.

National Society to Prevent Blindness
500 East Remington Road
Schaumburg, IL 60173
(312) 843-2020

Library, Large-Print, Recorded, and Transcription Services

The following resources provide reading materials made accessible by enlarging the print size, recording on cassette tape, or by translation into braille. Most of the materials are available at little or no cost to the borrower with low vision.

American Bible Society

This organization publishes and distributes the Bible in braille, large print, and in recorded formats.

American Bible Society
1865 Broadway
New York, NY 10023
(212) 581-7400

Bible Alliance, Inc.

This organization will provide a Bible on cassette tape upon request to anyone unable to read a print version. Although there is no charge for this service, a cassette talking book machine (available on a loan basis at no charge) from the Library of Congress should be obtained for listening to the taped Bible.

Bible Alliance, Inc.
P.O. Box 1549
Bradenton, FL 33506
(813) 748-3031

Jewish Braille Institute of America

This organization publishes large-print, recorded, and braille religious materials in Hebrew and English.

Jewish Braille Institute of America
110 East 13th Street
New York, NY 10016
(212) 889-2525

Library Reproduction Service

This company can enlarge the type size of print material from any book. The print is photographically reproduced, enlarged, printed, and bound in a library-quality hardcover. Favorite cookbooks, technical materials, charts and graphs, and foreign language material may all be put into the size of print requested by the reader.

Library Reproduction Service
1977 South Los Angeles Street
Los Angeles, CA 90011-1096
(213) 749-2463
(800) 255-5002

National Library Services for the Blind and Physically Handicapped (NLS)

In cooperation with a network of regional and subregional libraries, the National Library Service for the Blind and Physically Handicapped provides a free library service to persons who are unable to use standard printed material because of visual or physical disabilities. Books and magazines in recorded form (Talking Books) and in braille are delivered to eligible readers by postage-free mail and can be returned in the same manner. Specially designed phonographs and cassette players are also loaned free of charge to persons who borrow talking books from the library. Contact your local library or state services for the blind for an application and information.

National Library Services for the Blind
and Physically Handicapped (NLS)
Library Of Congress
1291 Taylor Street, N.W.
Washington, DC 20542
(202) 707-5100
(202) 707-0712 FAX

The Canadian National Institute for the Blind Library for the Blind

The CNIB Library for the Blind is the Canadian equivalent of the library.

The Canadian National Institute for the Blind
Library for the Blind
1929 Bayview Avenue
Toronto, ON M4G 3E8
Canada
(416) 480-7520

M. C. Migel Memorial Library

This specialized library has a comprehensive collection of written materials on blindness and low vision. Not a medical library, but rather a collection of publications about blindness and people who are blind. A bibliography of the subjects available may be obtained on request.

M. C. Migel Memorial Library
American Foundation for the Blind
15 West 16th Street
New York, NY 10011
(212) 620-2000
(800) 232-5463

Reader's Digest Large-Print Edition

The large-print version of the popular publication is available by contacting the publisher.

Reader's Digest Large-Print Edition
P.O. Box 241
Mt. Morris, IL 61054
(815) 734-6963

New York Times Large Type Weekly

The large-print version of the popular weekly publication, including the crossword puzzle, is available by contacting the publisher.

New York Times Large Type Weekly
New York Times Company
229 West 43rd Street
New York, NY 10036

Recording for the Blind

This nonprofit service provides educational and professional books and other materials for people who have low vision or are blind, and are unable to read standard print educational materials. Cassette books are loaned and books on computer diskette may also be purchased. There is a lifetime registration fee of $25.

Recording for the Blind
20 Roszel Road
Princeton, NJ 08540
(800) 221–4792 (for book orders and inquiries)
(609) 452–0606
FAX (609) 987–8116

G. K. Hall & Co.

This company sells unabridged best sellers (popular fiction, romances, mysteries, and westerns) and nonfiction (references, anthologies, and cookbooks) in comfortable large print, both hardcover and paperback. Call for a free "Large-Print-Books-By-Mail" catalog.

G. K. Hall & Co.
100 Front Street, Box 500
Riverside, NJ 08075-7500
(800) 257–5755 (For orders and inquiries)
(800) 343–2806 (For catalog requests)
(617) 423–3990 (For catalog requests in Alaska, Hawaii, and Massachusetts)

Education

The following organization provides educational services for people who are blind or visually impaired.

Hadley School for the Blind

This correspondence school for adults offers classes in a wide variety of subjects. The lessons are mailed on audio cassette tape or in braille and assignments are returned via mail.

Hadley School for the Blind
700 Elm Street
Winnetka, IL 60093
(800) 323-4238
(312) 446-8111

Recreation

American Blind Bowling Association

This association promotes bowling games and tournaments for people who are blind. A list of local and state associations is available by contacting the national office.

American Blind Bowling Association
3500 Terry Drive
Norfolk, VA 23518
(804) 857-7267

Blind Outdoor Leisure Development (BOLD)

BOLD, a national organization with many local affiliates, promotes recreational activities and opportunities for people who are blind or have visual impairments. BOLD provides instruction in the skills needed by sighted guides for recreational activities. While BOLD began as an organization to promote skiing for people who are blind, the activities some of their affiliates sponsor include canoeing, camping, and tandem bicycling.

Blind Outdoor Leisure Development (BOLD)
533 East Main Street
Aspen, CO 81611
(303) 925-8922

Ski For Light, Inc.

This not-for-profit organization was founded in 1975 to promote physical fitness and social well-being for blind and mobility-impaired adults. Training is provided to volunteer instructor/guides to assist with recreational downhill and cross country skiing for people who are blind or visually impaired. An annual ski weekend is sponsored.

Ski For Light, Inc.
1455 West Lake Street
Minneapolis, MN 55408
(612) 827-3232

Other

Descriptive Video Services (DVS)

Descriptive Video Services (DVS) is a system allowing a separate audio broadcast as part of a television transmission. A separate commentary provides a descriptive translation of the regular program. Facial expressions, the physical setting, body movements, and other visual aspects are described. To find out more about DVS, the needed equipment, or to get a list of stations that have the broadcast available, contact WGBH.

Descriptive Video Services (DVS)
WGBH
125 Western Avenue
Boston, MA 02134
(617) 492-2777

Rehabilitation Research and Training Center on Blindness and Low Vision

A national center conducting research and sponsoring conferences and workshops on the rehabilitation of people who are blind or have low vision.

Rehabilitation Research and Training Center on
Blindness and Low Vision
Mississippi State University
P.O. Drawer 6189
Mississippi State, MS 39762
(601) 325-2001

Appendix B

State and Provincial Services for the Blind

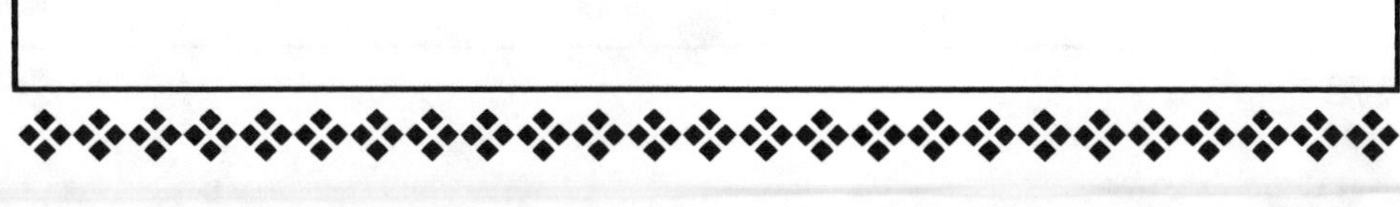

State Services for the Blind

Alabama

Division of Rehabilitation Services
P.O. Box 11586
Montgomery, AL 36111-0586
(205) 281–8780

Alaska

Division of Vocational Rehabilitation
Box F, MS 0581
Juneau, AK 99811–0500
(907) 465–2814

Arizona

Rehabilitation Services Administration
Department of Economic Security
1300 West Washington Street
Phoenix, AZ 85007
(602) 542–3332

Arkansas

Division of Services for the Blind
Department of Human Services
P.O. Box 3237
411 Victory Street
Little Rock, AR 72203
(501) 371–2587

California

Department of Rehabilitation
830 K Street Mall
Sacramento, CA 95814
(916) 445-3971

Colorado

Rehabilitation Services
Department of Social Services
1575 Sherman Street, 4th Floor
Denver, CO 80203-1741
(303) 866-5196

District of Columbia

D. C. Rehabilitation Services
Government of the District of Columbia
605 G Street, N.W., Room 1101
Washington, DC 20001
(202) 727-3227

Connecticut

Board of Education & Services for the Blind
Department of Human Resources
170 Ridge Road
Wethersfield, CT 06109
(203) 566-5800

Delaware

Division for the Visually Impaired
Biggs Building
Health & Social Service Campus
1901 North DuPont Highway
New Castle, DE 19720
(302) 421-5730

Florida

Division of Blind Services
Department of Education
2540 Executive Center Circle, West
Douglas Building
Tallahassee, FL 32301
(904) 488-1330

Georgia

Division of Rehabilitation Services
Department of Human Resources
878 Peachtree Street, N.E., Room 706
Atlanta, GA 30309
(404) 894-6670

Hawaii

Division of Vocational Rehabilitation
Department of Human Services
Bishop Trust Building
1000 Bishop Street, Room 615
Honolulu, HI 96813
(808) 548-4769

Idaho

Idaho Commission for the Blind
341 West Washington Street
Boise, ID 83702
(208) 334–3220

Illinois

Illinois Department of Rehabilitation Services
623 East Adams Street
P.O. Box 19429
Springfield, IL 62794-9429
(217) 782–2093

Indiana

Division of Rehabilitation Services
Indiana Department of Human Services
P.O. Box 7083
ISTA Building
150 West Market Street
Indianapolis, IN 46207-7083
(317) 232–1147

Iowa

Department for the Blind
524 4th Street
Des Moines, IA 50309-2364
(515) 281–7986

Kansas

Rehabilitation Services
Department of Social & Rehabilitation Services
300 Southwest Oakley Street
Biddle Building, 1st Floor
Topeka, KS 66606
(913) 296-3911

Kentucky

Kentucky Department for the Blind
427 Versailles Road
Frankfort, KY 40601
(502) 564-4754

Louisiana

Division of Rehabilitation Services
Department of Social Services
P.O. Box 94371
Baton Rouge, LA 70804
(504) 342-2285

Maine

Bureau of Rehabilitation
Department of Human Services
35 Anthony Avenue
Augusta, ME 04333-0011
(207) 289-2266

Maryland

Division of Vocational Rehabilitation
Administrative Offices
2301 Argonne Drive
Baltimore, MD 21218
(301) 554–3000

Massachusetts

Massachusetts Commission for the Blind
88 Kingston Street
Boston, MA 02111-2227
(617) 727–5550

Michigan

Commission for the Blind
Department of Labor
201 North Washington Square
Lansing, MI 48909
(517) 373–2062

Minnesota

State Services for the Blind
1745 University Avenue
St. Paul, MN 55104
(612) 642–0508

Mississippi

Division of Vocational Rehabilitation for the Blind
P.O. Box 4872
Jackson, MS 39215
(601) 354-6411

Missouri

Bureau for the Blind
Division of Family Services
619 East Capitol
Jefferson City, MO 65101
(314) 751-4249

Montana

Department of Social & Rehabilitation Services
Rehabilitation/Visual Services Division
P.O. Box 4210
111 Sanders
Helena, MT 59604
(406) 444-2590

Nebraska

Services for the Visually Impaired
Department of Public Institutions
4600 Valley Road
Lincoln, NB 68510-4844
(402) 471-2891

Nevada

Rehabilitation Division
Department of Human Resources
505 East King Street, 5th Floor
Carson City, NV 90710
(702) 687-4440

New Hampshire

Division of Vocational Rehabilitation
State Department of Education
78 Regional Drive
Concord, NH 03301-9686
(603) 271-3471

New Jersey

Commission for the Blind and Visually Impaired
P.O. Box 47017
153 Halsey Street
Newark, NJ 07102
(201) 648-2324

New Mexico

Commission for the Blind
Pera Building, Room 205
Santa Fe, NM 87503
(505) 827-4479

New York

State Department of Social Services
Commission for the Blind & Visually Handicapped
10 Eyck Office Building
40 North Pearl Street
Albany, NY 12243
(518) 473–1801

North Carolina

Division of Services for the Blind
Department of Human Resources
309 Ashe Avenue
Raleigh, NC 27606
(919) 733–9822

North Dakota

Office of Vocational Rehabilitation
Department of Human Service
State Capitol
600 East Boulevard Avenue
Bismarck, ND 58505-0295
(701) 224–2907

Oklahoma

Rehabilitation Services Division
Department of Human Services
2409 North Kelley
Oklahoma City, OK 73125
(405) 424–6006, Ext. 2840

Ohio

Ohio Rehabilitation Services Commission
400 East Campus View Boulevard
Columbus, OH 43235-4604
(614) 438–1210

Oregon

Commission for the Blind
535 S.E. 12th Avenue
Portland, OR 97214
(503) 238–8375

Pennsylvania

Bureau of Blindness & Visual Services
Department of Public Welfare
1301 North 7th Street
P.O. Box 2675
Harrisburg, PA 17105
(717) 787–6176

Rhode Island

Rhode Island States Services for the
Blind & Visually Impaired
Department of Human Services
275 Westminster Street, 5th Floor
Providence, RI 02903
(401) 277–2300

South Carolina

Commission for the Blind
1430 Confederate Avenue
Columbia, SC 29201
(803) 734–7520

South Dakota

Division of Service to the Blind & Visually Impaired
700 North Governors Drive
Pierre, SD 57501-2275
(605) 773–4644

Texas

Texas Commission for the Blind
Administration Building
4800 North Lamar Boulevard
Austin, TX 78711
(512) 459–2600

Utah

Utah State Office of Rehabilitation
250 East 500 South
Salt Lake City, UT 84111
(801) 538–7530

Vermont

Vermont Division for the Blind & Visually Impaired
Agency of Human Services
Osgood Building, Waterbury Complex
103 South Main Street
Waterbury, VT 05676
(802) 241–2211

Virginia

Virginia Department for the Visually Handicapped
Commonwealth of Virginia
397 Azalea Avenue
Richmond, VA 23227-3697
(804) 371–3145

Washington

Department of Services for the Blind
521 East Legion Way, MS: FD-11
Olympia, WA 98504-1422
(206) 586–1224

West Virginia

Division of Rehabilitation Services
State Board of Rehabilitation
State Capitol Complex
Charleston, WV 25305
(304) 766–4601

Wisconsin

Division of Vocational Rehabilitation
Office for the Blind
1 West Wilson Street, 8th Floor
P.O. Box 7852
Madison, WI 53707
(608) 266-1281

Wyoming

Division of Vocational Rehabilitation
Department of Employment
1100 Herschler Building
Cheyenne, WY 82002
(307) 777-7385

Canadian Provincial Services for the Blind

The Canadian National Institute for the Blind (CNIB)
National Office
1931 Bayview Avenue
Toronto, ON
M4G 4C8
(416) 480-7580

British Columbia — Yukon Division

350 East 36th Avenue
Vancouver, BC
V5W 1C6
(604) 321-2311

Alberta — Northwest Territories Division

12010 Jasper Avenue
Edmonton, AB
T5K 0P3
(403) 488–4871

Saskatchewan Division

2550 Broad Street
Regina, SK
S4P 3Z4
(306) 525–2571

Manitoba Division

1080 Portage Avenue
Winnipeg, MB
R3G 3M3
(204) 774–5421

Ontario Division

1929 Bayview Avenue
Toronto, ON
M4G 3E8
(416) 486–2500

Quebec Division

1010, rue Ste-Catherine Est
Suite P-100
Montreal, PQ
H2L 2G3
(514) 284–2040

New Brunswick Division

231 Saunders Street
Fredericton, NB
E3B 1N6
(506) 458-0060

Nova Scotia — Prince Edward Island Division

6136 Almon Street
Halifax, NS
B3K 1T8
(902) 453-1480

Newfoundland and Labrador Division

70 The Boulevard
St. John's, NF
A1A 1K2
(709) 754-1180

CNIB Library for the Blind

1929 Bayview Avenue
Toronto, ON
M4G 3E8
(416) 480-7520

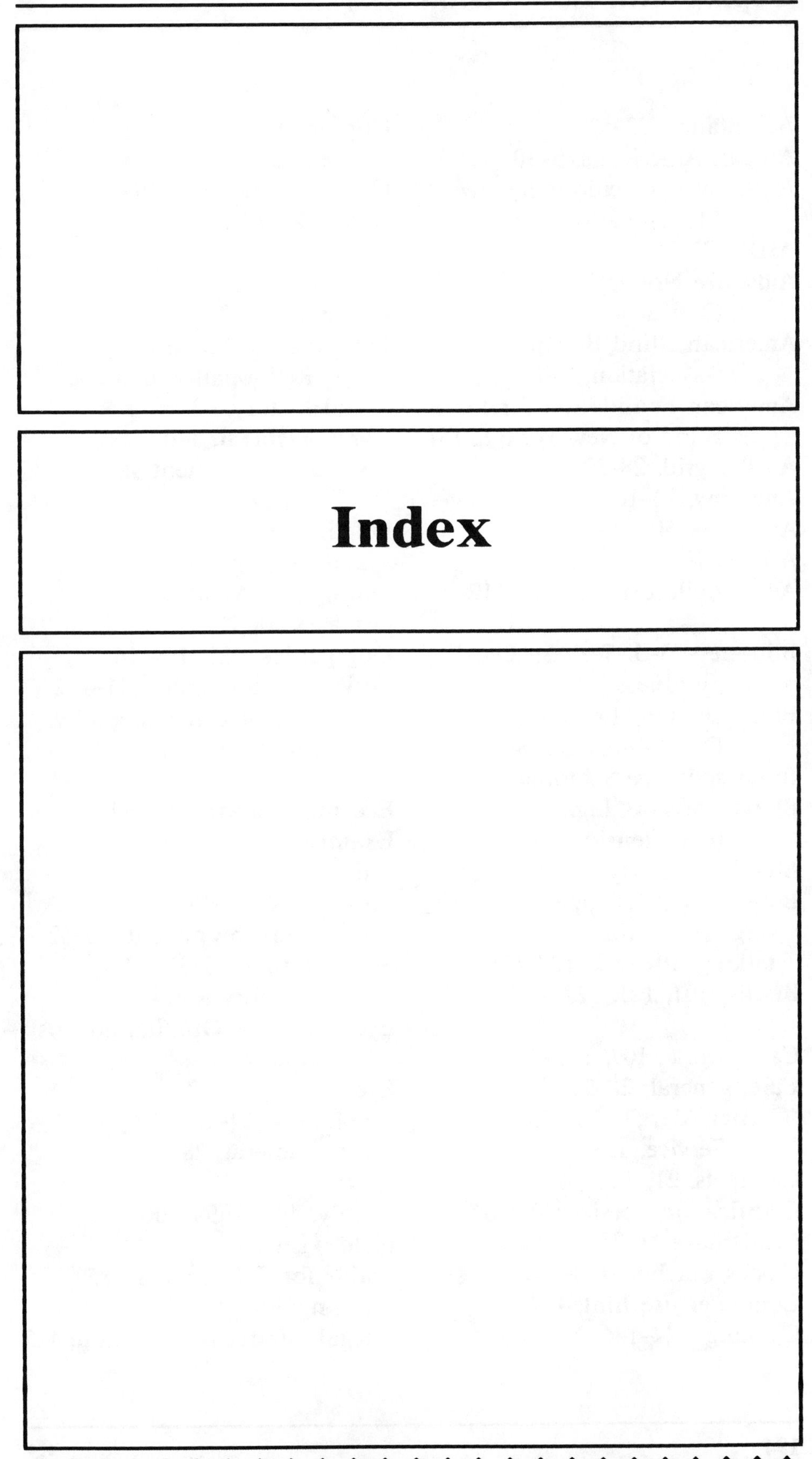

Index